KAPLAN
CLASSICS OF
MEDICINE

The

CORPUS

HIPPOCRATES

FOREWORD BY CONRAD FISCHER M.D.

KAPLAN
PUBLISHING
New York

Foreword by Dr. Conrad Fischer © 2008

Published by Kaplan Publishing, a division of Kaplan, Inc.
1 Liberty Plaza, 24th Floor
New York, NY 10006

Printed in the United States of America

August 2008

10 9 8 7 6 5 4 3 2 1

ISBN-13: 978-1-4277-9798-8

CONTENTS

FOREWORD

"Practice two things....either help, or do not harm." Imagine a world organized according to this teaching of the ancient Greek philosopher Hippocrates. Imagine every person as embodying this principle. Extraordinary!

How little we must think of this simple idea! Not much of the world around us—nations, armies, economies, and technology—follows the notion "Help, or do not harm."

In an extraordinary moment during the fourth century BCE, a philosopher declared that the personal and professional lives of the physician were to be ordered from this principle. It seems ridiculously obvious.

Yet in 1999, the Institute of Medicine of the United States estimated that medical errors caused anywhere from 44,000 to 98,000 deaths per year in the United States. That's at least as many as the number who die each year from suicide or motor vehicle accidents and many multiples more than those who die from AIDS or tuberculosis in the United States. Many of these unnecessary deaths stem from the failure to adhere to the advice "do not harm." Hippocrates devised this standard of behavior, which seems obvious. But 25 centuries later, our society has not fulfilled simple principles like "I won't hurt you," "I will only do what I know," and "I will not participate in torture." The major obstacle to understanding *The Corpus* is, I believe, the false conviction that the medical profession and our greater society already function under these precepts.

In *The Corpus*, Hippocrates says, "Although the art of healing is the most noble of all the arts, yet, because of the ignorance both of its professors and of their rash critics it has at this time fallen into the least repute of them all." Couldn't this have been written on the front page of today's *New York Times*? Let us for a moment consider what it was like to learn from Hippocrates in his time and ask if his teachings remain pertinent, timely, and shockingly current. Imagine a time without lawyers, courts, and the licensing we doctors take for granted. What controls human behavior in the absence of external control? Only the personal integrity of the individual. In the "Hippocratic Oath," Hippocrates has us swear, "I will use my power to help the sick to the best of my ability and judgment." As a patient, would you prefer that a physician be discouraged from harming you by fear of punishment or by his own personal integrity? A doctor's honor compels her to do what is right simply because it is right. We look for the same integrity in everyone from our plumber and our accountant to the leaders we elect. We seek the type of person who swears, "Whatever I see or hear, professionally or privately, which ought not to be divulged, I will keep secret and tell no one."

Hippocrates wrote: "Vita brevis, ars longa," or "Life is short, and the art is long." He, along with his students, created the first reproducible literature on disease. Before Hippocrates, even the most diligent practitioner had only had the benefit of his single lifetime of experience. Now we have the observations and organized thought of thousands of practitioners. Now we can advance knowledge and our profession.

We live in a sea of information, and we take for granted what was shatteringly new in the ancient world. Hippocrates was first to observe, describe, write, and create debate on the best way to advance his profession and medical science. Here we find ancient yet startlingly accurate depictions of malaria, meningitis, mumps, osteomyelitis, and pneumonia—a genuine breakthrough, the very concept of creating an organized, codified description of disease.

This breakthrough led to a new understanding of the physical nature of illnesses that had seemed supernatural in origin. In reading "The Sacred Disease," doctors should find nothing so delightful as reading the how the view of disease as divine intervention was confronted. His contemporaries saw illnesses like epilepsy and seizures as the will of the gods; Hippocrates says, "I do not believe that the 'Sacred disease' is any more divine or sacred than any other disease, but on the contrary has specific characteristics and a definite cause...It has been regarded as a divine visitation by those who, being only human, view it with ignorance and astonishment."

These observations represent a quintessential fork in the road in human history. Here, Hippocrates separates religion and belief from observable phenomena, subject to investigation and, ultimately, controllable. Again, you may ask yourself if this is obvious—yet you can turn on your television and watch prominent figures explain that hurricanes, floods, and even diseases like AIDS are God's divine retribution for earthly sin. Millions tune in, write checks, and believe. Read Hippocrates, and you'll find his rebuttal: "It is my opinion that those who first called this disease 'sacred' were the sort of people we now call witch-doctors, faith-healers, quacks, and charlatans....the people who *pretend* to be very pious and to be particularly wise."

We seek power. Through medical science, we seek the power to control and eliminate human disease and suffering; simultaneously as doctors, we seek the power to act with integrity and honor in both our ordinary days and times of extraordinary stress. In this quest, Hippocrates is our superman. His words offer the willpower of reason over superstition, championing evidence over belief and heroically defending rational observation, debate, and investigation against dogma and hypertrophied religiosity. Hippocrates declared us free from fear of the capricious visitations of dark spirits: "Human bodies cannot be polluted by a god...the presence of a god would be more likely to purify and sanctify than pollute it." In short, Hippocrates gives you, his reader, the power to think for yourself.

Even today, such audacity is breathtaking! Hippocrates seems to call to us from 2,500 years ago and ask that we act with the highest integrity in both our personal and professional lives. And he is as relevant in this moment as when he wrote what you will soon begin to read.

As you read *The Corpus,* I invite you to consider that "Help... or do not harm" remains the indispensible and central principle of modern medicine. Let us embody this idea and insist on it from all we meet, treat, and teach.

THE OATH OF HIPPOCRATES

I SWEAR by Apollo the physician, and Aesculapius, and Health, and All-heal, and all the gods and goddesses, that, according to my ability and judgment, I will keep this Oath and this stipulation—to reckon him who taught me this Art equally dear to me as my parents, to share my substance with him, and relieve his necessities if required; to look upon his offspring in the same footing as my own brothers, and to teach them this art, if they shall wish to learn it, without fee or stipulation; and that by precept, lecture, and every other mode of instruction, I will impart a knowledge of the Art to my own sons, and those of my teachers, and to disciples bound by a stipulation and oath according to the law of medicine, but to none others.

I will follow that system of regimen which, according to my ability and judgment, I consider for the benefit of my patients, and abstain from whatever is deleterious and mischievous.

I will give no deadly medicine to any one if asked, nor suggest any such counsel; and in like manner I will not give to a woman a pessary to produce abortion.

With purity and with holiness I will pass my life and practice my Art.

I will not cut persons laboring under the stone, but will leave this to be done by men who are practitioners of this work.

Into whatever houses I enter, I will go into them for the benefit of the sick, and will abstain from every voluntary act of mischief and corruption; and, further from the seduction of females or males, of freemen and slaves.

Whatever, in connection with my professional practice or not, in connection with it, I see or hear, in the life of men, which ought not to be spoken of abroad, I will not divulge, as reckoning that all such should be kept secret.

While I continue to keep this Oath unviolated, may it be granted to me to enjoy life and the practice of the art, respected by all men, in all times! But should I trespass and violate this Oath, may the reverse be my lot!

THE LAW

MEDICINE is of all the Arts the most noble; but, not with-standing, owing to the ignorance of those who practice it, and of those who, inconsiderately, form a judgment of them, it is at present far behind all the other arts. Their mistake appears to me to arise principally from this, that in the cities there is no punishment connected with the practice of medicine (and with it alone) except disgrace, and that does not hurt those who are familiar with it. Such persons are like the figures which are introduced in tragedies, for as they have the shape, and dress, and personal appearance of an actor, but are not actors, so also physicians are many in title but very few in reality.

2. Whoever is to acquire a competent knowledge of medi-cine, ought to be possessed of the following advantages: a natu-ral disposition; instruction; a favorable position for the study; early tuition; love of labor; leisure. First of all, a natural talent is required; for, when Nature opposes, everything else is in vain; but when Nature leads the way to what is most excellent, instruction in the art takes place, which the student must try to appropriate to himself by reflection, becoming an early pupil in a place well adapted for instruction. He must also bring to the task a love of labor and perseverance, so that the instruction taking root may bring forth proper and abundant fruits.

3. Instruction in medicine is like the culture of the produc-tions of the earth. For our natural disposition is, as it were, the soil; the tenets of our teacher are, as it were, the seed; instruction in youth is like the planting of the seed in the ground at the proper season; the place where the instruction is communicated is like the food imparted to vegetables by the atmosphere; diligent study is like the cultivation of the fields; and it is time which imparts strength to all things and brings them to maturity.

4. Having brought all these requisites to the study of medicine, and having acquired a true knowledge of it, we shall thus, in traveling through the cities, be esteemed physicians not only in name but in reality. But inexperience is a bad treasure, and a bad fund to those who possess it, whether in opinion or reality, being devoid of self-reliance and contentedness, and the nurse both of timidity and audacity. For timidity betrays a want of powers, and audacity a want of skill. There are, indeed, two things, knowledge and opinion, of which the one makes its possessor really to know, the other to be ignorant.

5. Those things which are sacred, are to be imparted only to sacred persons; and it is not lawful to import them to the profane until they have been initiated in the mysteries of the science.

ON ANCIENT
MEDICINE

WHOEVER having undertaken to speak or write on Medicine, have first laid down for themselves some hypothesis to their argument, such as hot, or cold, or moist, or dry, or whatever else they choose (thus reducing their subject within a narrow compass, and supposing only one or two original causes of diseases or of death among mankind), are all clearly mistaken in much that they say; and this is the more reprehensible as relating to an art which all men avail themselves of on the most important occasions, and the good operators and practitioners in which they hold in especial honor. For there are practitioners, some bad and some far otherwise, which, if there had been no such thing as Medicine, and if nothing had been investigated or found out in it, would not have been the case, but all would have been equally unskilled and ignorant of it, and everything concerning the sick would have been directed by chance. But now it is not so; for, as in all the other arts, those who practise them differ much from one another in dexterity and knowledge, so is it in like manner with Medicine. Wherefore I have not thought that it stood in need of an empty hypothesis, like those subjects which are occult and dubious, in attempting to handle which it is necessary to use some hypothesis; as, for example, with regard to things above us and things below the earth; if any one should treat of these and undertake to declare how they are constituted, the reader or hearer could not find out, whether what is delivered be true or false; for there is nothing which can be referred to in order to discover the truth.

2. But all these requisites belong of old to Medicine, and an origin and way have been found out, by which many and elegant discoveries have been made, during a length of time, and others will yet be found out, if a person possessed of the proper ability, and knowing those discoveries which have been made, should proceed from them to prosecute his investigations. But whoever, rejecting and despising all these, attempts to pursue another course and form of inquiry, and says he has discovered anything, is deceived himself and deceives others, for the thing is impossible. And for what reason it is impossible, I will now endeavor to explain, by stating and showing what the art really is. From this it will be manifest that discoveries cannot possibly be made in any other way. And most especially, it appears to me, that whoever treats of this art should treat of things which are familiar to the common people. For of nothing else will such a one have to inquire or treat, but of the diseases under which the common people have labored, which diseases and the causes of their origin and departure, their increase and decline, illiterate persons cannot easily find out themselves, but still it is easy for them to understand these things when discovered and expounded by others. For it is nothing more than that every one is put in mind of what had occurred to himself. But whoever does not reach the capacity of the illiterate vulgar and fails to make them listen to him, misses his mark. Wherefore, then, there is no necessity for any hypothesis.

3. For the art of Medicine would not have been invented at first, nor would it have been made a subject of investigation (for there would have been no need of it), if when men are indisposed, the same food and other articles of regimen which they eat and drink when in good health were proper for them, and if no others were preferable to these. But now necessity itself made medicine to be sought out and discovered by men, since the same things when administered to the sick, which agreed with them when in good health, neither did nor do agree with them. But to go still further back, I hold that the diet and food which people in health now use would not have been discovered, provided it had suited with man to eat and drink in like manner as the ox, the horse, and all other animals, except man, do of the productions of the earth, such as fruits, weeds, and grass; for from such things these animals grow, live free of disease, and require no other kind of food. And, at first, I am of opinion that man used the same sort of food, and that the present articles of diet had been discovered and invented only after a long lapse of time, for when they suffered much and severely from strong and brutish diet, swallowing things which were raw, unmixed, and possessing great strength, they became exposed to strong pains and diseases, and to early deaths. It is likely, indeed, that from habit they would suffer less from these things then than we would now, but still they would suffer severely even then; and it is likely that the greater number, and those who had weaker constitutions, would all perish; whereas the stronger would hold out for a longer time, as even nowadays some, in consequence of using strong articles of food, get off with little trouble, but others with much pain and suffering. From this necessity it appears to me that they would search out the food befitting their nature, and thus discover that which we now use: and that from wheat, by macerating it, stripping it of its hull, grinding it all down, sifting, toasting, and baking it, they formed bread; and from barley they formed cake (maza), performing many operations in regard to it;

they boiled, they roasted, they mixed, they diluted those things which are strong and of intense qualities with weaker things, fashioning them to the nature and powers of man, and considering that the stronger things Nature would not be able to manage if administered, and that from such things pains, diseases, and death would arise, but such as Nature could manage, that from them food, growth, and health, would arise. To such a discovery and investigation what more suitable name could one give than that of Medicine? since it was discovered for the health of man, for his nourishment and safety, as a substitute for that kind of diet by which pains, diseases, and deaths were occasioned.

4. And if this is not held to be an art, I do not object. For it is not suitable to call any one an artist of that which no one is ignorant of, but which all know from usage and necessity. But still the discovery is a great one, and requiring much art and investigation. Wherefore those who devote themselves to gymnastics and training, are always making some new discovery, by pursuing the same line of inquiry, where, by eating and drinking certain things, they are improved and grow stronger than they were.

5. Let us inquire then regarding what is admitted to be Medicine; namely, that which was invented for the sake of the sick, which possesses a name and practitioners, whether it also seeks to accomplish the same objects, and whence it derived its origin. To me, then, it appears, as I said at the commencement, that nobody would have sought for medicine at all, provided the same kinds of diet had suited with men in sickness as in good health. Wherefore, even yet, such races of men as make no use of medicine, namely, barbarians, and even certain of the Greeks, live in the same way when sick as when in health; that is to say, they take what suits their appetite, and neither abstain from, nor restrict themselves in anything for which they have a desire. But

those who have cultivated and invented medicine, having the same object in view as those of whom I formerly spoke, in the first place, I suppose, diminished the quantity of the articles of food which they used, and this alone would be sufficient for certain of the sick, and be manifestly beneficial to them, although not to all, for there would be some so affected as not to be able to manage even small quantities of their usual food, and as such persons would seem to require something weaker, they invented soups, by mixing a few strong things with much water, and thus abstracting that which was strong in them by dilution and boiling. But such as could not manage even soups, laid them aside, and had recourse to drinks, and so regulated them as to mixture and quantity, that they were administered neither stronger nor weaker than what was required.

6. But this ought to be well known, that soups do not agree with certain persons in their diseases, but, on the contrary, when administered both the fevers and the pains are exacerbated, and it becomes obvious that what was given has proved food and increase to the disease, but a wasting and weakness to the body. But whatever persons so affected partook of solid food, or cake, or bread, even in small quantity, would be ten times and more decidedly injured than those who had taken soups, for no other reason than from the strength of the food in reference to the affection; and to whomsoever it is proper to take soups and not eat solid food, such a one will be much more injured if he eat much than if he eat little, but even little food will be injurious to him. But all the causes of the sufferance refer themselves to this rule, that the strongest things most especially and decidedly hurt man, whether in health or in disease.

7. What other object, then, had he in view who is called a physician, and is admitted to be a practitioner of the art, who found out the regimen and diet befitting the sick, than he who originally found out and prepared for all mankind that kind of food which we all now use, in place of the former savage and brutish mode of living? To me it appears that the mode is the same, and the discovery of a similar nature. The one sought to abstract those things which the constitution of man cannot digest, because of their wildness and intemperature, and the other those things which are beyond the powers of the affection in which any one may happen to be laid up. Now, how does the one differ from the other, except that the latter admits of greater variety, and requires more application, whereas the former was the commencement of the process?

8. And if one would compare the diet of sick persons with that of persons in health, he will find it not more injurious than that of healthy persons in comparison with that of wild beasts and of other animals. For, suppose a man laboring under one of those diseases which are neither serious and unsupportable, nor yet altogether mild, but such as that, upon making any mistake in diet, it will become apparent, as if he should eat bread and flesh, or any other of those articles which prove beneficial to healthy persons, and that, too, not in great quantity, but much less than he could have taken when in good health; and that another man in good health, having a constitution neither very feeble, nor yet strong, eats of those things which are wholesome and strengthening to an ox or a horse, such as vetches, barley, and the like, and that, too, not in great quantity, but much less than he could take; the healthy person who did so would be subjected to no less disturbance and danger than the sick person who took bread or cake unseasonably. All these things are proofs that Medicine is to be prosecuted and discovered by the same method as the other.

9. And if it were simply, as is laid down, that such things as are stronger prove injurious, but such as are weaker prove beneficial and nourishing, both to sick and healthy persons, it were an easy matter, for then the safest rule would be to circumscribe the diet to the lowest point. But then it is no less mistake, nor one that injuries a man less, provided a deficient diet, or one consisting of weaker things than what mare proper, be administered. For, in the constitution of man, abstinence may enervate, weaken, and kill. And there are many other ills, different from those of repletion, but no less dreadful, arising from deficiency of food; wherefore the practice in those cases is more varied, and requires greater accuracy. For one must aim at attaining a certain measure, and yet this measure admits neither weight nor calculation of any kind, by which it may be accurately determined, unless it be the sensation of the body; wherefore it is a task to learn this accurately, so as not to commit small blunders either on the one side or the other, and in fact I would give great praise to the physician whose mistakes are small, for perfect accuracy is seldom to be seen, since many physicians seem to me to be in the same plight as bad pilots, who, if they commit mistakes while conducting the ship in a calm do not expose themselves, but when a storm and violent hurricane overtake them, they then, from their ignorance and mistakes, are discovered to be what they are, by all men, namely, in losing their ship. And thus bad and commonplace physicians, when they treat men who have no serious illness, in which case one may commit great mistakes without producing any formidable mischief (and such complaints occur much more frequently to men than dangerous ones): under these circumstances, when they commit mistakes, they do not expose themselves to ordinary men; but when they fall in with a great, a strong, and a dangerous disease, then their mistakes and want of skill are made apparent to all. Their punishment is not far off, but is swift in overtaking both the one and the other.

10. And that no less mischief happens to a man from unseasonable depletion than from repletion, may be clearly seen upon reverting to the consideration of persons in health. For, to some, with whom it agrees to take only one meal in the day, and they have arranged it so accordingly; whilst others, for the same reason, also take dinner, and this they do because they find it good for them, and not like those persons who, for pleasure or from any casual circumstance, adopt the one or the other custom and to the bulk of mankind it is of little consequence which of these rules they observe, that is to say, whether they make it a practice to take one or two meals. But there are certain persons who cannot readily change their diet with impunity; and if they make any alteration in it for one day, or even for a part of a day, are greatly injured thereby. Such persons, provided they take dinner when it is not their wont, immediately become heavy and inactive, both in body and mind, and are weighed down with yawning, slumbering, and thirst; and if they take supper in addition, they are seized with flatulence, tormina, and diarrhea, and to many this has been the commencement of a serious disease, when they have merely taken twice in a day the same food which they have been in the custom of taking once. And thus, also, if one who has been accustomed to dine, and this rule agrees with him, should not dine at the accustomed hour, he will straightway feel great loss of strength, trembling, and want of spirits, the eyes of such a person will become more pallid, his urine thick and hot, his mouth bitter; his bowels will seem, as it were, to hang loose; he will suffer from vertigo, lowness of spirit, and inactivity,— such are the effects; and if he should attempt to take at supper the same food which he was wont to partake of at dinner, it will appear insipid, and he will not be able to take it off; and these things, passing downwards with tormina and rumbling, burn up his bowels; he experiences insomnolency or troubled and disturbed dreams; and to many of them these symptoms are the commencement of some disease.

11. But let us inquire what are the causes of these things which happened to them. To him, then, who was accustomed to take only one meal in the day, they happened because he did not wait the proper time, until his bowels had completely derived benefit from and had digested the articles taken at the preceding meal, and until his belly had become soft, and got into a state of rest, but he gave it a new supply while in a state of heat and fermentation, for such bellies digest much more slowly, and require more rest and ease. And as to him who had been accustomed to dinner, since, as soon as the body required food, and when the former meal was consumed, and he wanted refreshment, no new supply was furnished to it, he wastes and is consumed from want of food. For all the symptoms which I describe as befalling to this man I refer to want of food. And I also say that all men who, when in a state of health, remain for two or three days without food, experience the same unpleasant symptoms as those which I described in the case of him who had omitted to take dinner.

12. Wherefore, I say, that such constitutions as suffer quickly and strongly from errors in diet, are weaker than others that do not; and that a weak person is in a state very nearly approaching to one in disease; but a person in disease is the weaker, and it is, therefore, more likely that he should suffer if he encounters anything that is unseasonable. It is difficult, seeing that there is no such accuracy in the Art, to hit always upon what is most expedient, and yet many cases occur in medicine which would require this accuracy, as we shall explain. But on that account, I say, we ought not to reject the ancient Art, as if it were not, and had not been properly founded, because it did not attain accuracy in all things, but rather, since it is capable of reaching to the greatest exactitude by reasoning, to receive it and admire its discoveries, made from a state of great ignorance, and as having been well and properly made, and not from chance.

13. But I wish the discourse to revert to the new method of those who prosecute their inquiries in the Art by hypothesis. For if hot, or cold, or moist, or dry, be that which proves injurious to man, and if the person who would treat him properly must apply cold to the hot, hot to the cold, moist to the dry, and dry to the moist—let me be presented with a man, not indeed one of a strong constitution, but one of the weaker, and let him eat wheat, such as it is supplied from the thrashing-floor, raw and unprepared, with raw meat, and let him drink water. By using such a diet I know that he will suffer much and severely, for he will experience pains, his body will become weak, and his bowels deranged, and he will not subsist long. What remedy, then, is to be provided for one so situated? Hot? or cold? or moist? or dry? For it is clear that it must be one or other of these. For, according to this principle, if it is one of the which is injuring the patient, it is to be removed by its contrary. But the surest and most obvious remedy is to change the diet which the person used, and instead of wheat to give bread, and instead of raw flesh, boiled, and to drink wine in addition to these; for by making these changes it is impossible but that he must get better, unless completely disorganized by time and diet. What, then, shall we say? whether that, as he suffered from cold, these hot things being applied were of use to him, or the contrary? I should think this question must prove a puzzler to whomsoever it is put. For whether did he who prepared bread out of wheat remove the hot, the cold, the moist, or the dry principle in it?—for the bread is consigned both to fire and to water, and is wrought with many things, each of which has its peculiar property and nature, some of which it loses, and with others it is diluted and mixed.

14. And this I know, moreover, that to the human body it makes a great difference whether the bread be fine or coarse; of wheat with or without the hull, whether mixed with much or little water, strongly wrought or scarcely at all, baked or raw—and a multitude of similar differences; and so, in like manner, with the cake (maza); the powers of each, too, are great, and the one nowise like the other. Whoever pays no attention to these things, or, paying attention, does not comprehend them, how can he understand the diseases which befall a man? For, by every one of these things, a man is affected and changed this way or that, and the whole of his life is subjected to them, whether in health, convalescence, or disease. Nothing else, then, can be more important or more necessary to know than these things. So that the first inventors, pursuing their investigations properly, and by a suitable train of reasoning, according to the nature of man, made their discoveries, and thought the Art worthy of being ascribed to a god, as is the established belief. For they did not suppose that the dry or the moist, the hot or the cold, or any of these are either injurious to man, or that man stands in need of them, but whatever in each was strong, and more than a match for a man's constitution, whatever he could not manage, that they held to be hurtful, and sought to remove. Now, of the sweet, the strongest is that which is intensely sweet; of the bitter, that which is intensely bitter; of the acid, that which is intensely acid; and of all things that which is extreme, for these things they saw both existing in man, and proving injurious to him. For there is in man the bitter and the salt, the sweet and the acid, the sour and the insipid, and a multitude of other things having all sorts of powers both as regards quantity and strength. These, when all mixed and mingled up with one another, are not apparent, neither do they hurt a man; but when any of them is separate, and stands by itself, then it becomes perceptible, and hurts a man. And thus, of articles of food, those which are unsuitable and hurtful to man when administered, every one is either bitter, or intensely so, or saltish or acid, or something else intense and strong, and therefore we are disordered by them in like manner as we are by the secretions in the body. But all those things which a man eats and drinks are devoid of any such intense and well-marked quality, such as bread, cake, and many other things of a similar nature which man is accustomed to use for food, with the exception of condiments and confectioneries, which are made to gratify the palate and for luxury. And from those things, when received into the body abundantly, there is no disorder nor dissolution of the powers belonging to the body; but strength, growth, and nourishment result from them, and this for no other reason than because they are well mixed, have nothing in them of an immoderate character, nor anything strong, but the whole forms one simple and not strong substance.

15. I cannot think in what manner they who advance this doctrine, and transfer Art from the cause I have described to hypothesis, will cure men according to the principle which they have laid down. For, as far as I know, neither the hot nor the cold, nor the dry, nor the moist, has ever been found unmixed with any other quality; but I suppose they use the same articles of meat and drink as all we other men do. But to this substance they give the attribute of being hot, to that cold, to that dry, and to that moist. Since it would be absurd to advise the patient to take something hot, for he would straightway ask what it is? so that he must either play the fool, or have recourse to some one of the well known substances; and if this hot thing happen to be sour, and that hot thing insipid, and this hot thing has the power of raising a disturbance in the body (and there are many other kinds of heat, possessing many opposite powers), he will be obliged to administer some one of them, either the hot and the sour, or the hot and the insipid, or that which, at the same time, is cold and sour (for there is such a substance), or the cold and the insipid. For, as I think, the very opposite effects will result from either of these, not only in man, but also in a bladder, a vessel of wood, and in many other things possessed of far less sensibility than man; for it is not the heat which is possessed of great efficacy, but the sour and the insipid, and other qualities as described by me, both in man and out of man, and that whether eaten or drunk, rubbed in externally, and otherwise applied.

16. But I think that of all the qualities heat and cold exercise the least operation in the body, for these reasons: as long time as hot and cold are mixed up with one another they do not give trouble, for the cold is attempered and rendered more moderate by the hot, and the hot by the cold; but when the one is wholly separate from the other, then it gives pain; and at that season when cold is applied it creates some pain to a man, but quickly, for that very reason, heat spontaneously arises in him without requiring any aid or preparation. And these things operate thus both upon men in health and in disease. For example, if a person in health wishes to cool his body during winter, and bathes either in cold water or in any other way, the more he does this, unless his body be fairly congealed, when he resumes his clothes and comes into a place of shelter, his body becomes more heated than before. And thus, too, if a person wish to be warmed thoroughly either by means of a hot bath or strong fire, and straightway having the same clothing on, takes up his abode again in the place he was in when he became congealed, he will appear much colder, and more disposed to chills than before. And if a person fan himself on account of a suffocating heat, and having procured refrigeration for himself in this manner, cease doing so, the heat and suffocation will be ten times greater in his case than in that of a person who does nothing of the kind. And, to give a more striking example, persons travelling in the snow, or otherwise in rigorous weather, and contracting great cold in their feet, their hands, or their head, what do they not suffer from inflammation and tingling when they put on warm clothing and get into a hot place? In some instances, blisters arise as if from burning with fire, and they do not suffer from any of those unpleasant symptoms until they become heated. So readily does either of these pass into the other; and I could mention many other examples. And with regard to the sick, is it not in those who experience a rigor that the most acute fever is apt to break out? And yet not so strongly neither, but that it ceases in a short time, and, for the most part, without having occasioned much mischief; and while it remains, it is hot, and passing over the whole body, ends for the most part in the feet, where the chills and cold were most intense and lasted longest; and, when sweat supervenes, and the fever passes off, the patient is much colder than if he had not taken the fever at all. Why then should that which so quickly passes into the opposite extreme, and loses its own powers spontaneously, be reckoned a mighty and serious affair? And what necessity is there for any great remedy for it?

17. One might here say—but persons in ardent fevers, pneumonia, and other formidable diseases, do not quickly get rid of the heat, nor experience these rapid alterations of heat and cold. And I reckon this very circumstance the strongest proof that it is not from heat simply that men get into the febrile state, neither is it the sole cause of the mischief, but that this species of heat is bitter, and that acid, and the other saltish, and many other varieties; and again there is cold combined with other qualities. These are what proves injurious; heat, it is true, is present also, possessed of strength as being that which conducts, is exacerbated and increased along with the other, but has no power greater than what is peculiar to itself.

18. With regard to these symptoms, in the first place those are most obvious of which we have all often had experience. Thus, then, in such of us as have a coryza and defluxion from the nostrils, this discharge is much more acrid than that which formerly was formed in and ran from them daily; and it occasions swelling of the nose, and it inflames, being of a hot and extremely ardent nature, as you may know, if you apply your hand to the place; and, if the disease remains long, the part becomes ulcerated although destitute of flesh and hard; and the heat in the nose ceases, not when the defluxion takes place and the inflammation is present, but when the running becomes thicker and less acrid, and more mixed with the former secretion, then it is that the heat ceases. But in all those cases in which this decidedly proceeds from cold alone, without the concourse of any other quality, there is a change from cold to hot, and from hot to cold, and these quickly supervene, and require no coction. But all the others being connected, as I have said, with acrimony and intemperance of humors, pass off in this way by being mixed and concocted.

19. But such defluxions as are determined to the eyes being possessed of strong and varied acrimonies, ulcerate the eyelids, and in some cases corrode the parts below the eyes upon which they flow, and even occasion rupture and erosion of the tunic which surrounds the eyeball. But pain, heat, and extreme burning prevail until the defluxions are concocted and become thicker, and concretions form about the eyes, and the coction takes place from the fluids being mixed up, diluted, and digested together. And in defluxions upon the throat, from which are formed hoarseness, cynanche, crysipelas, and pneumonia, all these have at first saltish, watery, and acrid discharges, and with these the diseases gain strength. But when the discharges become thicker, more concocted, and are freed from all acrimony, then, indeed, the fevers pass away, and the other symptoms which annoyed the patient; for we must account those things the cause of each complaint, which, being present in a certain fashion, the complaint exists, but it ceases when they change to another combination. But those which originate from pure heat or cold, and do not participate in any other quality, will then cease when they undergo a change from cold to hot, and from hot to cold; and they change in the manner I have described before. Wherefore, all the other complaints to which man is subject arise from powers (qualities?). Thus, when there is an overflow of the bitter principle, which we call yellow bile, what anxiety, burning heat, and loss of strength prevail! but if relieved from it, either by being purged spontaneously, or by means of a medicine seasonably administered, the patient is decidedly relieved of the pains and heat; but while these things float on the stomach, unconcocted and undigested, no contrivance could make the pains and fever cease; and when there are acidities of an acrid and aeruginous character, what varieties of frenzy, gnawing pains in the bowels and chest, and inquietude, prevail! and these do not cease until the acidities be purged away, or are calmed down and mixed with other fluids. The coction, change, attenuation, and thickening into the form of humors, take place through many and various forms; therefore the crises and calculations of time are of great importance in such matters; but to all such changes hot and cold are but little exposed, for these are neither liable to putrefaction nor thickening. What then shall we say of the change? that it is a combination (crasis) of these humors having different powers toward one another. But the hot does not loose its heat when mixed with any other thing except the cold; nor again, the cold, except when mixed with the hot. But all other things connected with man become the more mild and better in proportion as they are mixed with the more things besides. But a man is in the best possible state when they are concocted and at rest, exhibiting no one peculiar quality; but I think I have said enough in explanation of them.

20. Certain sophists and physicians say that it is not possible for any one to know medicine who does not know what man is [and how he was made and how constructed], and that whoever would cure men properly, must learn this in the first place. But this saying rather appertains to philosophy, as Empedocles and certain others have described what man in his origin is, and how he first was made and constructed. But I think whatever such has been said or written by sophist or physician concerning nature has less connection with the art of medicine than with the art of painting. And I think that one cannot know anything certain respecting nature from any other quarter than from medicine; and that this knowledge is to be attained when one comprehends the whole subject of medicine properly, but not until then; and I say that this history shows what man is, by what causes he was made, and other things accurately. Wherefore it appears to me necessary to every physician to be skilled in nature, and strive to know, if he would wish to perform his duties, what man is in relation to the articles of food and drink, and to his other occupations, and what are the effects of each of them to every one. And it is not enough to know simply that cheese is a bad article of food, as disagreeing with whoever eats of it to satiety, but what sort of disturbance it creates, and wherefore, and with what principle in man it disagrees; for there are many other articles of food and drink naturally bad which affect man in a different manner. Thus, to illustrate my meaning by an example, undiluted wine drunk in large quantity renders a man feeble; and everybody seeing this knows that such is the power of wine, and the cause thereof; and we know, moreover, on what parts of a man's body it principally exerts its action; and I wish the same certainty to appear in other cases. For cheese (since we used it as an example) does not prove equally injurious to all men, for there are some who can take it to satiety without being hurt by it in the least, but, on the contrary, it is wonderful what strength it imparts to those it agrees with; but there are some who do not bear it well, their constitutions are different, and they differ in this respect, that what in their body is incompatible with cheese, is roused and put in commotion by such a thing; and those in whose bodies such a humor happens to prevail in greater quantity and intensity, are likely to suffer the more from it. But if the thing had been pernicious to of man, it would have hurt all. Whoever knows these things will not suffer from it.

21. During convalescence from diseases, and also in protracted diseases, many disorders occur, some spontaneously, and some from certain things accidentally administered. I know that the common herd of physicians, like the vulgar, if there happen to have been any innovation made about that day, such as the bath being used, a walk taken, or any unusual food eaten, all which were better done than otherwise, attribute notwithstanding the cause of these disorders, to some of these things, being ignorant of the true cause but proscribing what may have been very proper. Now this ought not to be so; but one should know the effects of a bath or a walk unseasonably applied; for thus there will never be any mischief from these things, nor from any other thing, nor from repletion, nor from such and such an article of food. Whoever does not know what effect these things produce upon a man, cannot know the consequences which result from them, nor how to apply them.

22. And it appears to me that one ought also to know what diseases arise in man from the powers, and what from the structures. What do I mean by this? By powers, I mean intense and strong juices; and by structures, whatever conformations there are in man. For some are hollow, and from broad contracted into narrow; some expanded, some hard and round, some broad and suspended, some stretched, some long, some dense, some rare and succulent, some spongy and of loose texture. Now, then, which of these figures is the best calculated to suck to itself and attract humidity from another body? Whether what is hollow and expanded, or what is solid and round, or what is hollow, and from broad, gradually turning narrow? I think such as from hollow and broad are contracted into narrow: this may be ascertained otherwise from obvious facts: thus, if you gape wide with the mouth you cannot draw in any liquid; but by protruding, contracting, and compressing the lips, and still more by using a tube, you can readily draw in whatever you wish. And thus, too, the instruments which are used for cupping are broad below and gradually become narrow, and are so constructed in order to suck and draw in from the fleshy parts. The nature and construction of the parts within a man are of a like nature; the bladder, the head, the uterus in woman; these parts clearly attract, and are always filled with a juice which is foreign to them. Those parts which are hollow and expanded are most likely to receive any humidity flowing into them, but cannot attract it in like manner. Those parts which are solid and round could not attract a humidity, nor receive it when it flows to them, for it would glide past, and find no place of rest on them. But spongy and rare parts, such as the spleen, the lungs, and the breasts, drink up especially the juices around them, and become hardened and enlarged by the accession of juices. Such things happen to these organs especially. For it is not with the spleen as with the stomach, in which there is a liquid, which it contains and evacuates every day; but when it (the spleen) drinks up and receives a fluid into itself, the hollow and lax parts of it are filled, even the small interstices; and, instead of being rare and soft, it becomes hard and dense, and it can neither digest nor discharge its contents: these things it suffers, owing to the nature of its structure. Those things which engender flatulence or tormina in the body, naturally do so in the hollow and broad parts of the body, such as the stomach and chest, where they produce rumbling noises; for when they do not fill the parts so as to be stationary, but have changes of place and movements, there must necessarily be noise and apparent movements from them. But such parts as are fleshy and soft, in these there occur torpor and obstructions, such as happen in apoplexy. But when it (the flatus?) encounters a broad and resisting structure, and rushes against such a part, and this happens when it is by nature not strong so as to be able to withstand it without suffering injury; nor soft and rare, so as to receive or yield to it, but tender, juicy, full of blood, and dense, like the liver, owing to its density and broadness, it resists and does not yield. But flatus, when it obtains admission, increases and becomes stronger, and rushes toward any resisting object; but owing to its tenderness, and the quantity of blood which it (the liver) contains, it cannot be without uneasiness; and for these reasons the most acute and frequent pains occur in the region of it, along with suppurations and chronic tumors (phymata). These symptoms also occur in the site of the diaphragm, but much less frequently; for the diaphragm is a broad, expanded, and resisting substance, of a nervous (tendinous?) and strong nature, and therefore less susceptible of pain; and yet pains and chronic abscesses do occur about it.

23. There are both within and without the body many other kinds of structure, which differ much from one another as to sufferings both in health and disease; such as whether the head be small or large; the neck slender or thick, long or short; the belly long or round; the chest and ribs broad or narrow; and many others besides, all which you ought to be acquainted with, and their differences; so that knowing the causes of each, you may make the more accurate observations.

24. And, as has been formerly stated, one ought to be acquainted with the powers of juices, and what action each of them has upon man, and their alliances towards one another. What I say is this: if a sweet juice change to another kind, not from any admixture, but because it has undergone a mutation within itself; what does it first become?—bitter? salt? austere? or acid? I think acid. And hence, an acid juice is the most improper of all things that can be administered in cases in which a sweet juice is the most proper. Thus, if one should succeed in his investigations of external things, he would be the better able always to select the best; for that is best which is farthest removed from that which is unwholesome.

THE BOOK OF
PROGNOSTICS

IT APPEARS to me a most excellent thing for the physician to cultivate Prognosis; for by foreseeing and foretelling, in the presence of the sick, the present, the past, and the future, and explaining the omissions which patients have been guilty of, he will be the more readily believed to be acquainted with the circumstances of the sick; so that men will have confidence to intrust themselves to such a physician. And he will manage the cure best who has foreseen what is to happen from the present state of matters. For it is impossible to make all the sick well; this, indeed, would have been better than to be able to foretell what is going to happen; but since men die, some even before calling the physician, from the violence of the disease, and some die immediately after calling him, having lived, perhaps, only one day or a little longer, and before the physician could bring his art to counteract the disease; it therefore becomes necessary to know the nature of such affections, how far they are above the powers of the constitution; and, moreover, if there be anything divine in the diseases, and to learn a foreknowledge of this also. Thus a man will be the more esteemed to be a good physician, for he will be the better able to treat those aright who can be saved, having long anticipated everything; and by seeing and announcing beforehand those who will live and those who will die, he will thus escape censure.

2. He should observe thus in acute diseases: first, the countenance of the patient, if it be like those of persons in health, and more so, if like itself, for this is the best of all; whereas the most opposite to it is the worst, such as the following; a sharp nose, hollow eyes, collapsed temples; the ears cold, contracted, and their lobes turned out: the skin about the forehead being rough, distended, and parched; the color of the whole face being green, black, livid, or lead-colored. If the countenance be such at the commencement of the disease, and if this cannot be accounted for from the other symptoms, inquiry must be made whether the patient has long wanted sleep; whether his bowels have been very loose; and whether he has suffered from want of food; and if any of these causes be confessed to, the danger is to be reckoned so far less; and it becomes obvious, in the course of a day and a night, whether or not the appearance of the countenance proceeded from these causes. But if none of these be said to exist, if the symptoms do not subside in the aforesaid time, it is to be known for certain that death is at hand. And, also, if the disease be in a more advanced stage either on the third or fourth day, and the countenance be such, the same inquiries as formerly directed are to be made, and the other symptoms are to be noted, those in the whole countenance, those on the body, and those in the eyes; for if they shun the light, or weep involuntarily, or squint, or if the one be less than the other, or if the white of them be red, livid, or has black veins in it; if there be a gum upon the eyes, if they are restless, protruding, or are become very hollow; and if the countenance be squalid and dark, or the color of the whole face be changed—all these are to be reckoned bad and fatal symptoms. The physician should also observe the appearance of the eyes from below the eyelids in sleep; for when a portion of the white appears, owing to the eyelids not being closed together, and when this is not connected with diarrhea or purgation from medicine, or when the patient does not sleep thus from habit, it is to be reckoned an unfavorable and very deadly symptom; but if the eyelid be contracted, livid, or pale, or also the lip, or nose, along with some of the other symptoms, one may know for certain that death is close at hand. It is a mortal symptom, also, when the lips are relaxed, pendent, cold, and blanched.

3. It is well when the patient is found by his physician reclining upon either his right or his left side, having his hands, neck, and legs slightly bent, and the whole body lying in a relaxed state, for thus the most of persons in health recline, and these are the best of postures which most resemble those of healthy persons. But to lie upon one's back, with the hands, neck, and the legs extended, is far less favorable. And if the patient incline forward, and sink down to the foot of the bed, it is a still more dangerous symptom; but if he be found with his feet naked and not sufficiently warm, and the hands, neck, and legs tossed about in a disorderly manner and naked, it is bad, for it indicates aberration of intellect. It is a deadly symptom, also, when the patient sleeps constantly with his mouth open, having his legs strongly bent and plaited together, while he lies upon his back; and to lie upon one's belly, when not habitual to the patient to sleep thus while in good health, indicates delirium, or pain in the abdominal regions. And for the patient to wish to sit erect at the acme of a disease is a bad symptom in all acute diseases, but particularly so in pneumonia. To grind the teeth in fevers, when such has not been the custom of the patient from childhood, indicates madness and death, both which dangers are to be announced beforehand as likely to happen; and if a person in delirium do this it is a very deadly symptom. And if the patient had an ulcer previously, or if one has occurred in the course of the disease, it is to be observed; for if the man be about to die the sore will become livid and dry, or yellow and dry before death.

4. Respecting the movement of the hands I have these observations to make: When in acute fevers, pneumonia, phrenitis, or headache, the hands are waved before the face, hunting through empty space, as if gathering bits of straw, picking the nap from the coverlet, or tearing chaff from the wall—all such symptoms are bad and deadly.

5. Respiration, when frequent, indicates pain or inflanunation in the parts above the diaphragm: a large respiration performed at a great interval announces delirium; but a cold respiration at nose or mouth is a very fatal symptom. Free respiration is to be looked upon as contributing much to the safety of the patient in all acute diseases, such as fevers, and those complaints which come to a crisis in forty days.

6. Those sweats are the best in all acute diseases which occur on the critical days, and completely carry off the fever. Those are favorable, too, which taking place over the whole body, show that the man is bearing the disease better. But those that do not produce this effect are not beneficial. The worst are cold sweats, confined to the head, face, and neck; these in an acute fever prognosticate death, or in a milder one, a prolongation of the disease; and sweats which occur over the whole body, with the characters of those confined to the neck, are in like manner bad. Sweats attended with a miliary eruption, and taking place about the neck, are bad; sweats in the form of drops and of vapour are good. One ought to know the entire character of sweats, for some are connected with prostration of strength in the body, and some with intensity of the inflammation.

7. That state of the hypochondrium is best when it is free from pain, soft, and of equal size on the right side and the left.

But if inflamed, or painful, or distended; or when the right and left sides are of disproportionate sizes;—all these appearances are to be dreaded. And if there be also pulsation in the hypochondrium, it indicates perturbation or delirium; and the physician should examine the eyes of such persons; for if their pupils be in rapid motion, such persons may be expected to go mad. A swelling in the hypochondrium, that is hard and painful, is very bad, provided it occupy the whole hypochondrium; but if it be on either side, it is less dangerous when on the left. Such swellings at the commencement of the disease prognosticate speedy death; but if the fever has passed twenty days, and the swelling has not subsided, it turns to a suppuration. A discharge of blood from the nose occurs to such in the first period, and proves very useful; but inquiry should be made if they have headache or indistinct vision; for if there be such, the disease will be determined thither. The discharge of blood is rather to be expected in those who are younger than thirty-five years. Such swellings as are soft, free from pain, and yield to the finger, occasion more protracted crises, and are less dangerous than the others. But if the fever continue beyond sixty days, without any subsidence of the swelling, it indicates that empyema is about to take place; and a swelling in any other part of the cavity will terminate in like manner. Such, then, as are painful, hard, and large, indicate danger of speedy death; but such as are soft, free of pain, and yield when pressed with the finger, are more chronic than these. Swellings in the belly less frequently form abscesses than those in the hypochondrium; and seldomest of all, those below the navel are converted into suppuration; but you may rather expect a hemorrhage from the upper parts. But the suppuration of all protracted swellings about these parts is to be anticipated. The collections of matter there are to be thus judged of: such as are determined outwards are the best when they are small, when they protrude very much, and swell to a point; such as are large and broad, and which do not swell out to a sharp point, are the worst. Of such as break internally, the best are those which have no external communication, but are covered and indolent; and when the whole place is free from discoloration. That pus is best which is white, homogeneous, smooth, and not at all fetid; the contrary to this is the worst.

8. All dropsies arising from acute diseases are bad; for they do not remove the fever, and are very painful and fatal. The most of them commence from the flanks and loins, but some from the liver; in those which derive their origin from the flanks and loins the feet swell, protracted diarrhoeas supervene, which neither remove the pains in the flanks and loins, nor soften the belly, but in dropsies which are connected with the liver there is a tickling cough, with scarcely any perceptible expectoration, and the feet swell; there are no evacuations from the bowels, unless such as are hard and forced; and there are swellings about the belly, sometimes on the one side and sometimes on the other, and these increase and diminish by turns.

9. It is a bad symptom when the head, hands, and feet are cold, while the belly and sides are hot; but it is a very good symptom when the whole body is equally hot. The patient ought to be able to turn round easily, and to be agile when raised up; but if he appear heavy in the rest of his body as well as in his hands and feet, it is more dangerous; and if, in addition to the weight, his nails and fingers become livid, immediate death may be anticipated; and if the hands and feet be black it is less dangerous than if they be livid, but the other symptoms must be attended, to; for if he appear to bear the illness well, and if certain of the salutary symptoms appear along with these there may be hope that the disease will turn to a deposition, so that the man may recover; but the blackened parts of the body will drop off. When the testicles and members are retracted upwards, they indicate strong pains and danger of death.

10. With regard to sleep—as is usual with us in health, the patient should wake during the day and sleep during the night. If this rule be anywise altered it is so far worse: but there will be little harm provided he sleep in the morning for the third part of the day; such sleep as takes place after this time is more unfavorable; but the worst of all is to get no sleep either night or day; for it follows from this symptom that the insomnolency is connected with sorrow and pains, or that he is about to become delirious.

11. The excrement is best which is soft and consistent, is passed at the hour which was customary to the patient when in health, in quantity proportionate to the ingests; for when the passages are such, the lower belly is in a healthy state. But if the discharges be fluid, it is favorable that they are not accompanied with a noise, nor are frequent, nor in great quantity; for the man being oppressed by frequently getting up, must be deprived of sleep; and if the evacuations be both frequent and large, there is danger of his falling into deliquium animi. But in proportion to the ingesta he should have evacuations twice or thrice in the day, once at night and more copiously in the morning, as is customary with a person in health. The faeces should become thicker when the disease is tending to a crisis; they ought to be yellowish and not very fetid. It is favorable that round worms be passed with the discharges when the disease is tending to a crisis. The belly, too, through the whole disease, should be soft and moderately distended; but excrements that are very watery, or white, or green, or very red, or frothy, are all bad. It is also bad when the discharge is small, and viscid, and white, and greenish, and smooth; but still more deadly appearances are the black, or fatty, or livid, or verdigris-green, or fetid. Such as are of varied characters indicate greater duration of the complaint, but are no less dangerous; such as those which resemble scrapings, those which are bilious, those resembling leeks, and the black; these being sometimes passed together, and sometimes singly. It is best when wind passes without noise, but it is better that flatulence should pass even thus than that it should be retained; and when it does pass thus, it indicates either that the man is in pain or in delirium, unless he gives vent to the wind spontaneously. Pains in the hypochondria, and swellings, if recent, and not accompanied with inflammation, are relieved by borborygmi supervening in the hypochondrium, more especially if it pass off with faeces, urine, and wind; but even although not, it will do good by passing along, and it also does good by descending to the lower part of the belly.

12. The urine is best when the sediment is white, smooth, and consistent during the whole time, until the disease come to a crisis, for it indicates freedom from danger, and an illness of short duration; but if deficient, and if it be sometimes passed clear, and sometimes with a white and smooth sediment, the disease will be more protracted, and not so void of danger. But if the urine be reddish, and the sediment consistent and smooth, the affection, in this case, will be more protracted than the former, but still not fatal. But farinaceous sediments in the urine are bad, and still worse are the leafy; the white and thin are very bad, but the furfuraceous are still worse than these. Clouds carried about in the urine are good when white, but bad if black. When the urine is yellow and thin, it indicates that the disease is unconcocted; and if it (the disease) should be protracted, there maybe danger lest the patient should not hold out until the urine be concocted. But the most deadly of all kinds of urine are the fetid, watery, black, and thick; in adult men and women the black is of all kinds of urine the worst, but in children, the watery. In those who pass thin and crude urine for a length of time, if they have otherwise symptoms of convalescence, an abscess may be expected to form in the parts below the diaphragm. And fatty substances floating on the surface are to be dreaded, for they are indications of melting. And one should consider respecting the kinds of urine, which have clouds, whether they tend upwards or downwards, and upwards or downwards, and the colors which they have and such as fall downwards, with the colors as described, are to be reckoned good and commended; but such as are carried upwards, with the colors as described, are to be held as bad, and are to be distrusted. But you must not allow yourself to be deceived if such urine be passed while the bladder is diseased; for then it is a symptom of the state, not of the general system, but of a particular viscus.

13. That vomiting is of most service which consists of phlegm and bile mixed together, and neither very thick nor in great quantity; but those vomitings which are more unmixed are worse. But if that which is vomited be of the color of leeks or livid, or black, whatever of these colors it be, it is to be reckoned bad; but if the same man vomit all these colors, it is to be reckoned a very fatal symptom. But of all the vomitings, the livid indicates the danger of death, provided it be of a fetid smell. But all the smells which are somewhat putrid and fetid, are bad in all vomitings.

14. The expectoration in all pains about the lungs and sides, should be quickly and easily brought up, and a certain degree of yellowness should appear strongly mixed up with the sputum. But if brought up long after the commencement of the pain, and of a yellow or ruddy color, or if it occasions much cough, or be not strongly mixed, it is worse; for that which is intensely yellow is dangerous, but the white, and viscid, and round, do no good. But that which is very green and frothy is bad; but if so intense as to appear black, it is still more dangerous than these; it is danger- ous than these; it is bad, if nothing is expectorated, and the lungs discharge nothing, but are gorged with matters which boil (as it were) in the air-passages. It is bad when coryza and sneezing either precede or follow affections of the lungs, but in all other affections, even the most deadly, sneezing is a salutary symp- tom. A yellow spittle mixed up with not much blood in cases of pneumonia, is salutary and very beneficial if spit up at the com- mencement of the disease, but if on the seventh day, or still later, it is less favorable. And all sputa are bad which do not remove the pain. But the worst is the black, as has been described. Of all others the sputa which remove the pain are the best.

15. When the pains in these regions do not cease, either with the discharge of the sputa, nor with alvine evacuations, nor from venesection, purging with medicine, nor a suitable regimen, it is to be held that they will terminate in suppurations. Of empye- mata such as are spit up while the sputum is still bilious, are very fatal, whether the bilious portion be expectorated separate, or along with the other; but more especially if the empyema begin to advance after this sputum on the seventh day of the disease. It is to be expected that a person with such an expectoration shall die on the fourteenth day, unless something favorable supervene. The following are favorable symptoms: to support the disease easily, to have free respiration, to be free from pain, to have the sputa readily brought up, the whole body to appear equally warm and soft, to have no thirst, the urine, and faeces, sleep, and sweats to be all favorable, as described before; when all these symptoms concur, the patient certainly will not die; but if some of these be present and some not, he will not survive longer than the fourteenth day. The bad symptoms are the opposite of these, namely, to bear the disease with difficulty, respiration large and dense, the pain not ceasing, the sputum scarcely coughed up, strong thirst, to have the body unequally affected by the febrile heat, the belly and sides intensely hot, the forehead, hands, and feet cold; the urine, and excrements, the sleep, and sweats, all bad, agreeably to the characters described above; if such a combination of symptoms accompany the expectoration, the man will certainly die before the fourteenth day, and either on the ninth or eleventh. Thus then one may conclude regarding this expectoration, that it is very deadly, and that the patient will not survive until the fourteenth day. It is by balancing the concomitant symptoms whether good or bad, that one is to form a prognosis; for thus it will most probably prove to be a true one. Most other suppurations burst, some on the twentieth, some on the thirtieth, some on the fortieth, and some as late as the sixtieth day.

16. One should estimate when the commencement of the suppuration will take place, by calculating from the day on which the patient was first seized with fever, or if he had a rigor, and if he says, that there is a weight in the place where he had pain formerly, for these symptoms occur in the commencement of suppurations. One then may expect the rupture of the abscesses to take place from these times according to the periods formerly stated. But if the empyema be only on either side, one should turn him and inquire if he has pain on the other side; and if the one side be hotter than the other, and when laid upon the sound side, one should inquire if he has the feeling of a weight hanging from above, for if so, the empyema will be upon the opposite side to that on which the weight was felt.

17. Empyema may be recognized in all cases by the following symptoms: In the first place, the fever does not go off, but is slight during the day, and increases at night, and copious sweats supervene, there is a desire to cough, and the patients expectorate nothing worth mentioning, the eyes become hollow, the cheeks have red spots on them, the nails of the hands are bent, the fingers are hot especially their extremities, there are swellings in the feet, they have no desire of food, and small blisters (phlyctaenae) occur over the body. These symptoms attend chronic empyemata, and may be much trusted to; and such as are of short standing are indicated by the same, provided they be accompanied by those signs which occur at the commencement, and if at the same time the patient has some difficulty of breathing. Whether they will break earlier or later may be determined by these symptoms; if there be pain at the commencement, and if the dyspnoea, cough, and ptyalism be severe, the rupture may be expected in the course of twenty days or still earlier; but if the pain be more mild, and all the other symptoms in proportion, you may expect from these the rupture to be later; but pain, dyspnoea, and ptyalism, must take place before the rupture of the abscess. Those patients recover most readily whom the fever leaves the same day that the abscess bursts,—when they recover their appetite speedily, and are freed from the thirst,—when the alvine discharges are small and consistent, the matter white, smooth, uniform in color, and free of phlegm, and if brought up without pain or strong coughing. Those die whom the fever does not leave, or when appearing to leave them it returns with an exacerbation; when they have thirst, but no desire of food, and there are watery discharges from the bowels; when the expectoration is green or livid, or pituitous and frothy; if all these occur they die, but if certain of these symptoms supervene, and others not, some patients die and some recover, after a long interval.

But from all the symptoms taken together one should form a judgment, and so in all other cases.

18. When abscesses form about the ears, after peripneumonic affections, or depositions of matter take place in the inferior extremities and end in fistula, such persons recover. The following observations are to be made upon them: if the fever persist, and the pain do not cease, if the expectoration be not normal, and if the alvine discharges be neither bilious, nor free and unmixed; and if the urine be neither copious nor have its proper sediment, but if, on the other hand, all the other salutary symptoms be present, in such cases abscesses may be expected to take place. They form in the inferior parts when there is a collection of phlegm about the hypochondria; and in the upper when the continue soft and free of pain, and when dyspnoea having been present for a certain time, ceases without any obvious cause. All deposits which take place in the legs after severe and dangerous attacks of pneumonia, are salutary, but the best are those which occur at the time when the sputa undergo a change; for if the swelling and pain take place while the sputa are changing from yellow and becoming of a purulent character, and are expectorated freely, under these circumstances the man will recover most favorably and the abscess becoming free of pain, will soon cease; but if the expectoration is not free, and the urine does not appear to have the proper sediment, there is danger lest the limb should be maimed, or that the case otherwise should give trouble. But if the abscesses disappear and go back, while expectoration does not take place, and fever prevails, it is a bad symptom; for there is danger that the man may get into a state of delirium and die. Of persons having empyema after peripneumonic affections, those that are advanced in life run the greatest risk of dying; but in the other kinds of empyema younger persons rather die. In cases of empyema treated by the cautery or incision, when the matter is pure, white, and not fetid, the patient recovers; but if of a bloody and dirty character, he dies.

19. Pains accompanied with fever which occur about the loins and lower parts, if they attack the diaphragm, and leave the parts below, are very fatal. Wherefore one ought to pay attention to the other symptoms, since if any unfavorable one supervene, the case is hopeless; but if while the disease is determined to the diaphragm, the other symptoms are not bad, there is great reason to expect that it will end in empyema. When the bladder is hard and painful, it is an extremely bad and mortal symptom, more especially in cases attended with continued fever; for the pains proceeding from the bladder alone are to kill the patient; and at such a time the bowels are not moved, or the discharges are hard and forced. But urine of a purulent character, and having a white and smooth sediment, relieves the patient. But if no amendment takes place in the characters of the urine, nor the bladder become soft, and the fever is of the continual type, it may be expected that the patient will die in the first stages of the complaint. This form attacks children more especially, from their seventh to their fifteenth year.

20. Fevers come to a crisis on the same days as to number on which men recover and die. For the mildest class of fevers, and those originating with the most favorable symptoms, cease on the fourth day or earlier; and the most malignant, and those setting in with the most dangerous symptoms, prove fatal on the fourth day or earlier. The first class of them as to violence ends thus: the second is protracted to the seventh day, the third to the eleventh, the fourth to the fourteenth, the fifth to the seventeenth, and the sixth to the twentieth. Thus these periods from the most acute disease ascend by fours up to twenty. But none of these can be truly calculated by whole days, for neither the year nor the months can be numbered by entire days. After these in the same manner, according to the same progression, the first period is of thirty-four days, the second of forty days, and the third of sixty days. In the commencement of these it is very difficult to determine those which will come to a crisis after a long interval; for these beginnings are very similar, but one should pay attention from the first day, and observe further at every additional tetrad, and then one cannot miss seeing how the disease will terminate. The constitution of quartans is agreeable to the same order. Those which will come to a crisis in the shortest space of time, are the easiest to be judged of; for the differences of them are greatest from the commencement, thus those who are going to recover breathe freely, and do not suffer pain, they sleep during the night, and have the other salutary symptoms, whereas those that are to die have difficult respiration, are delirious, troubled with insomnolency, and have other bad symptoms. Matters being thus, one may conjecture, according to the time, and each additional period of the diseases, as they proceed to a crisis. And in women, after parturition, the crises proceed agreeably to the same ratio.

21. Strong and continued headaches with fever, if any of the deadly symptoms be joined to them, are very fatal. But if without such symptoms the pain be prolonged beyond twenty days, a discharge of blood from the nose or some abscess in the inferior parts may be anticipated; but while the pain is recent, we may expect in like manner a discharge of blood from the nose, or a suppuration, especially if the pain be seated above the temples and forehead; but the hemorrhage is rather to be looked for in persons younger than thirty years, and the suppuration in more elderly persons.

22. Acute pain of the ear, with continual and strong fever, is to be dreaded; for there is danger that the man may become delirious and die. Since, then, this is a hazardous spot, one ought to pay particular attention to all these symptoms from the commencement. Younger persons die of this disease on the seventh day, or still earlier, but old persons much later; for the fevers and delirium less frequently supervene upon them, and on that account the ears previously come to a suppuration, but at these periods of life, relapses of the disease coming on generally prove fatal. Younger persons die before the ear suppurates; only if white matter run from the ear, there may be hope that a younger person will recover, provided any other favorable symptom be combined.

23. Ulceration of the throat with fever, is a serious affection, and if any other of the symptoms formerly described as being bad, be present, the physician ought to announce that his patient is in danger. Those quinsies are most dangerous, and most quickly prove fatal, which make no appearance in the fauces, nor in the neck, but occasion very great pain and difficulty of breathing; these induce suffocation on the first day, or on the second, the third, or the fourth. Such as, in like manner, are attended with pain, are swelled up, and have redness (erythema) in the throat, are indeed very fatal, but more protracted than the former, provided the redness be great. Those cases in which both the throat and the neck are red, are more protracted, and certain persons recover from them, especially if the neck and breast be affected with erythema, and the erysipelas be not determined inwardly. If neither the erysipelas disappear on the critical day, nor any abscess form outwardly, nor any pus be spit up, and if the patient fancy himself well, and be free from pain, death, or a relapse of the erythema is to be apprehended. It is much less hazardous when the swelling and redness are determined outwardly;

but if determined to the lungs, they superinduce delirium, and frequently some of these cases terminate in empyema. It is very dangerous to cut off or scarify enlarged uvulae while they and red and large, for inflammations and hemorrhages supervene; but one should try to reduce such swellings by some other means at this season. When the whole of it is converted into an abscess, which is called Uva, or when the extremity of the variety called Columella is larger and round, but the upper part thinner, at this time it will be safe to operate. But it will be better to open the bowels gently before proceeding to the operation, if time will permit, and the patient be not in danger of being suffocated.

24. When the fevers cease without any symptoms of resolution occurring, and not on the critical days, in such cases a relapse may be anticipated. When any of the fevers is protracted, although the man exhibits symptoms of recovery, and there is no longer pain from any inflammation, nor from any other visible cause, in such a case a deposit, with swelling and pain, may be expected in some one of the joints, and not improbably in those below. Such deposits occur more readily and in less time to persons under thirty years of age; and one should immediately suspect the formation of such a deposit, if the fever be protracted beyond twenty days; but to aged persons these less seldom happen, and not until the fever be much longer protracted. Such a deposit may be expected, when the fever is of a continual type, and that it will pass into a quartan, if it become intermittent, and its paroxysms come on in an irregular manner, and if in this form it approach autumn. As deposits form most readily in persons below thirty years of age, so quartans most commonly occur to persons beyond that age. It is proper to know that deposits occur most readily in winter, that then they are most protracted, but are less given to return. Whoever, in a fever that is not of a fatal character, says that he has pain in his head, and that some-thing dark appears to be before his eyes, and that he has pain at the stomach, will be seized with vomiting of bile; but if rigor also attack him, and the inferior parts of the hypochondrium are cold, vomiting is still nearer at hand; and if he eat or drink any-thing at such a season, it will be quickly vomited. In these cases, when the pain commences on the first day, they are particularly oppressed on the fourth and the fifth; and they are relieved on the seventh, but the greater part of them begin to have pain on the third day, and are most especially tossed on the fifth, but are relieved on the ninth or eleventh; but in those who begin to have pains on the fifth day, and other matters proceed properly with them, the disease comes to a crisis on the fourteenth day. But when in such a fever persons affected with headache, instead of having a dark appearance before their eyes, have dimness of vision, or flashes of light appear before their eyes, and instead of pain at the pit of the stomach, they have in their hypochon-drium a fullness stretching either to the right or left side, with-out either pain or inflammation, a hemorrhage from the nose is to be expected in such a case, rather than a vomiting. But it is in young persons particularly that the hemorrhage is to be expected, for in persons beyond the age of thirty-five, vomit-ings are rather to be anticipated. Convulsions occur to children if acute fever be present, and the belly be they cannot sleep, are agitated, and moan, and change color, and become green, livid, or ruddy. These complaints occur most readily to children which are very young up to their seventh year; older children and adults are not equally liable to be seized with convulsions in fevers, unless some of the strongest and worst symptoms precede, such as those which occur in frenzy. One must judge of children as of others, which will die and which recover, from the whole of the symptoms, as they have been specially described. These things I say respecting acute diseases, and the affections which spring from them.

25. He who would correctly beforehand those that will recover, and those that will die, and in what cases the disease will be protracted for many days, and in what cases for a shorter time, must be able to form a judgment from having made himself acquainted with all the symptoms, and estimating their powers in comparison with one another, as has been described, with regard to the others, and the urine and sputa, as when the patient coughs up pus and pus and bile together. One ought also to consider promptly the influx of epidemical diseases and the constitution of the season. One should likewise be well acquainted with the particular signs and the other symptoms, and not be ignorant how that, in every year, and at every season, bad symptoms prognosticate ill, and favorable symptoms good, since the aforesaid symptoms appear to have held true in Libya, in Delos, and in Scythia, from which it may be known that, in the same regions, there is no difficulty in attaining a knowledge of many more things than these; if having learned them, one knows also how to judge and reason correctly of them. But you should not complain because the name of any disease may happen not to be described here, for you may know all such as come to a crisis in the aforementioned times, by the same symptoms.

APHORISMS

SECTION I.

LIFE IS short, and Art long; the crisis fleeting; experience perilous, and decision difficult. The physician must not only be prepared to do what is right himself, but also to make the patient, the attendants, and externals cooperate.

2. In disorders of the bowels and vomitings, occurring spontaneously, if the matters purged be such as ought to be purged, they do good, and are well borne; but if not, the contrary. And so artificial evacuations, if they consist of such matters as should be evacuated, do good, and are well borne; but if not, the contrary. One, then, ought to look to the country, the season, the age, and the diseases in which they are proper or not.

3. In the athletae, embonpoint, if carried to its utmost limit, is dangerous, for they cannot remain in the same state nor be stationary; and since, then, they can neither remain stationary nor improve, it only remains for them to get worse; for these reasons the embonpoint should be reduced without delay, that the body may again have a commencement of reparation. Neither should the evacuations, in their case, be carried to an extreme, for this also is dangerous, but only to such a point as the person's constitution can endure. In like manner, medicinal evacuations, if carried to an extreme, are dangerous; and again, a restorative course, if in the extreme, is dangerous.

4. A slender restricted diet is always dangerous in chronic diseases, and also in acute diseases, where it is not requisite. And again, a diet brought to the extreme point of attenuation is dangerous; and repletion, when in the extreme, is also dangerous.

5. In a restricted diet, patients who transgress are thereby more hurt (than in any other?); for every such transgression, whatever it may be, is followed by greater consequences than in a diet somewhat more generous. On this account, a very slender, regulated, and restricted diet is dangerous to persons in health, because they bear transgressions of it more difficultly. For this reason, a slender and restricted diet is generally more dangerous than one a little more liberal.

6. For extreme diseases, extreme methods of cure, as to restriction, are most suitable.

7. When the disease is very acute, it is attended with extremely severe symptoms in its first stage; and therefore an extremely attenuating diet must be used. When this is not the case, but it is allowable to give a more generous diet, we may depart as far from the severity of regimen as the disease, by its mildness, is removed from the extreme.

8. When the disease is at its height, it will then be necessary to use the most slender diet.

9. We must form a particular judgment of the patient, whether he will support the diet until the acme of the disease, and whether he will sink previously and not support the diet, or the disease will give way previously, and become less acute.

10. In those cases, then, which attain their acme speedily, a restricted diet should be enjoined at first; but in those cases which reach their acme later, we must retrench at that period or a little before it; but previously we must allow a more generous diet to support the patient.

11. We must retrench during paroxysms, for to exhibit food would be injurious. And in all diseases having periodical paroxysms, we must restrict during the paroxysms.

12. The exacerbations and remissions will be indicated by the diseases, the seasons of the year, the reciprocation of the periods, whether they occur every day, every alternate day, or after a longer period, and by the supervening symptoms; as, for example, in pleuritic cases, expectoration, if it occur at the commencement, shortens the attack, but if it appear later, it prolongs the same; and in the same manner the urine, and alvine discharges, and sweats, according as they appear along with favorable or unfavorable symptoms, indicate diseases of a short or long duration.

13. Old persons endure fasting most easily; next, adults; young persons not nearly so well; and most especially infants, and of them such as are of a particularly lively spirit.

14. Growing bodies have the most innate heat; they therefore require the most food, for otherwise their bodies are wasted. In old persons the heat is feeble, and therefore they require little fuel, as it were, to the flame, for it would be extinguished by much. On this account, also, fevers in old persons are not equally acute, because their bodies are cold.

15. In winter and spring the bowels are naturally the hottest, and the sleep most prolonged; at these seasons, then, the most sustenance is to be administered; for as the belly has then most innate heat, it stands in need of most food. The well-known facts with regard to young persons and the athletae prove this.

16. A humid regimen is befitting in all febrile diseases, and particularly in children, and others accustomed to live on such a diet.

17. We must consider, also, in which cases food is to be given once or twice a day, and in greater or smaller quantities, and at intervals. Something must be conceded to habit, to season, to country, and to age.

18. Invalids bear food worst during summer and autumn, most easily in winter, and next in spring.

19. Neither give nor enjoin anything to persons during periodical paroxysms, but abstract from the accustomed allowance before the crisis.

20. When things are at the crisis, or when they have just passed it, neither move the bowels, nor make any innovation in the treatment, either as regards purgatives or any other such stimulants, but let things alone.

21. Those things which require to be evacuated should be evacuated, wherever they most tend, by the proper outlets.

22. We must purge and move such humors as are concocted, not such as are unconcocted, unless they are struggling to get out, which is mostly not the case.

23. The evacuations are to be judged of not by their quantity, but whether they be such as they should be, and how they are borne. And when proper to carry the evacuation to deliquium animi, this also should be done, provided the patient can support it.

24. Use purgative medicines sparingly in acute diseases, and at the commencement, and not without proper circumspection.

25. If the matters which are purged be such as should be purged, the evacuation is beneficial, and easily borne; but, not withstanding, if otherwise, with difficulty.

SECTION II.

1. In whatever disease sleep is laborious, it is a deadly symptom; but if sleep does good, it is not deadly.

2. When sleep puts an end to delirium, it is a good symptom.

3. Both sleep and insomnolency, when immoderate, are bad.

4. Neither repletion, nor fasting, nor anything else, is good when more than natural.

5. Spontaneous lassitude indicates disease.

6. Persons who have a painful affection in any part of the body, and are in a great measure sensible of the pain, are disordered in intellect.

7. Those bodies which have been slowly emaciated should be slowly recruited; and those which have been quickly emaciated should be quickly recruited.

8. When a person after a disease takes food, but does not improve in strength, it indicates that the body uses more food than is proper; but if this happen when he does not take food, it is to be understood evacuation is required.

9. When one wishes to purge, he should put the body into a fluent state.

10. Bodies not properly cleansed, the more you nourish the more you injure.

11. It is easier to fill up with drink than with food.

12. What remains in diseases after the crisis is apt to produce relapses.

13. Persons in whom a crisis takes place pass the night preceding the paroxysm uncomfortably, but the succeeding night generally more comfortably.

14. In fluxes of the bowels, a change of the dejections does good, unless the change be of a bad character.

15. When the throat is diseased, or tubercles (phymata) form on the body, attention must paid to the secretions; for if they be bilious, the disease affects the general system; but if they resemble those of a healthy person, it is safe to give nourishing food.

16. When in a state of hunger, one ought not to undertake labor.

17. When more food than is proper has been taken, it occasions disease; this is shown by the treatment.

18. From food which proves nourishing to the body either immediately or shortly, the dejections also are immediate.

19. In acute diseases it is not quite safe to prognosticate either death or recovery.

20. Those who have watery discharges from their bowels when young have dry when they are old; and those who have dry discharges when they are young will have watery when they are old.

21. Drinking strong wine cures hunger.

22. Diseases which arise from repletion are cured by depletion; and those that arise from depletion are cured by repletion; and in general, diseases are cured by their contraries.

23. Acute disease come to a crisis in fourteen days.

24. The fourth day is indicative of the seventh; the eighth is the commencement of the second week; and hence, the eleventh being the fourth of the second week, is also indicative; and again, the seventeenth is indicative, as being the fourth from the fourteenth, and the seventh from the eleventh.

25. The summer quartans are, for the most part, of short duration; but the autumnal are protracted, especially those occurring near the approach of winter.

26. It is better that a fever succeed to a convulsion, than a convulsion to a fever.

27. We should not trust ameliorations in diseases when they are not regular, nor be much afraid of bad symptoms which occur in an irregular form; for such are commonly inconstant, and do not usually continue, nor have any duration.

28. In fevers which are not altogether slight, it is a bad symptom for the body to remain without any diminution of bulk, or to be wasted beyond measure; for the one state indicates a protracted disease, and the other weakness of body.

29. If it appear that evacuations are required, they should be made at the commencement of diseases; at the acme it is better to be quiet.

30. Toward the commencement and end of diseases all the symptoms are weaker, and toward the acme they are stronger.

31. When a person who is recovering from a disease has a good appetite, but his body does not improve in condition, it is a bad symptom.

32. For the most part, all persons in ill health, who have a good appetite at the commencement, but do not improve, have a bad appetite again toward the end; whereas, those who have a very bad appetite at the commencement, and afterward acquire a good appetite, get better off.

33. In every disease it is a good sign when the patient's intellect is sound, and he is disposed to take whatever food is offered to him; but the contrary is bad.

34. In diseases, there is less danger when the disease is one to which the patient's constitution, habit, age, and the season are allied, than when it is one to which they are not allied.

35. In all diseases it is better that the umbilical and hypogastric regions preserve their fullness; and it is a bad sign when they are very slender and emaciated; in the latter case it is dangerous to administer purgatives.

36. Persons in good health quickly lose their strength by taking purgative medicines, or using bad food.

37. Purgative medicines agree ill with persons in good health.

38. An article of food or drink which is slightly worse, but more palatable, is to be preferred to such as are better but less palatable.

39. Old have fewer complaints than young; but those chronic diseases which do befall them generally never leave them.

40. Catarrhs and coryza in very old people are not concocted.

41. Persons who have had frequent and severe attacks of swooning, without any manifest cause, die suddenly.

42. It is impossible to remove a strong attack of apoplexy, and not easy to remove a weak attack.

43. Of persons who have been suspended by the neck, and are in a state of insensibility, but not quite dead, those do not recover who have foam at the mouth.

44. Persons who are naturally very fat are apt to die earlier than those who are slender.

45. Epilepsy in young persons is most frequently removed by changes of air, of country, and of modes of life.

46. Of two pains occurring together, not in the same part of the body, the stronger weakens the other.

47. Pains and fevers occur rather at the formation of pus than when it is already formed.

48. In every movement of the body, whenever one begins to endure pain, it will be relieved by rest.

49. Those who are accustomed to endure habitual labors, although they be weak or old, bear them better than strong and young persons who have not been so accustomed.

50. Those things which one has been accustomed to for a long time, although worse than things which one is not accustomed to, usually give less disturbance; but a change must sometimes be made to things one is not accustomed to.

51. To evacuate, fill up, heat, cool, or otherwise, move the body in any way much and suddenly, is dangerous; and whatever is excessive is inimical to nature; but whatever is done by little and little is safe, more especially when a transition is made from one thing to another.

52. When doing everything according to indications, although things may not turn out agreeably to indication, we should not change to another while the original appearances remain.

53. Those persons who have watery discharges from the bowels when they are young, come off better than those who have dry; but in old age they come off worse, for the bowels in aged persons are usually dried up.

54. Largeness of person in youth is noble and not unbecoming; but in old age it is inconvenient, and worse than a smaller structure.

SECTION III.

1. The changes of the season mostly engender diseases, and in the seasons great changes either of heat or of cold, and the rest agreeably to the same rule.

2. Of natures (temperaments?), some are well—or ill-adapted for summer, and some for winter.

3. Of diseases and ages, certain of them are well—or ill-adapted to different seasons, places, and kinds of diet.

4. In the seasons, when during the same day there is at one time heat and at another time cold, the diseases of autumn may be expected.

5. South winds induce dullness of hearing, dimness of visions, heaviness of the head, torpor, and languor; when these prevail, such symptoms occur in diseases. But if the north wind prevail, coughs, affections of the throat, hardness of the bowels, dysuria attended with rigors, and pains of the sides and breast occur. When this wind prevails, all such symptoms may be expected in diseases.

6. When summer is like spring, much sweating may be expected in fevers.

7. Acute diseases occur in droughts; and if the summer be particularly such, according to the constitution which it has given to the year, for the most part such diseases maybe expected.

8. In seasons which are regular, and furnish the productions of the season at the seasonable time, the diseases are regular, and come readily to a crisis; but in inconstant seasons, the diseases are irregular, and come to a crisis with difficulty.

9. In autumn, diseases are most acute, and most mortal, on the whole. The spring is most healthy, and least mortal.

10. Autumn is a bad season for persons in consumption.

11. With regard to the seasons, if the winter be of a dry and northerly character, and the spring rainy and southerly, in summer there will necessarily be acute fevers, ophthalmies, and dysenteries, especially in women, and in men of a humid temperament.

12. If the but the spring dry and northerly, women whose term of delivery should be in spring, have abortions from any slight cause; and those who reach their full time, bring forth children who are feeble, and diseased, so that they either die presently, or, if they live, are puny and unhealthy. Other people are subject to dysenteries and ophthalmies, and old men to catarrhs, which quickly cut them off.

13. If the summer be dry and northerly and the autumn rainy and southerly, headaches occur in winter, with coughs, hoarsenesses, coryzae, and in some cases consumptions.

14. But if the autumn be northerly and dry, it agrees well with persons of a humid temperament, and with women; but others will be subject to dry ophthalmies, acute fevers, coryzae, and in some cases melancholy.

15. Of the constitutions of the year, the dry, upon the whole, are more healthy than the rainy, and attended with less mortality.

16. The diseases which occur most frequently in rainy seasons are, protracted fevers, fluxes of the bowels, mortifications, epilepsies, apoplexies, and quinsies; and in dry, consumptive diseases, ophthalmies, arthritic diseases, stranguries, and dysenteries.

17. With regard to the states of the weather which continue but for a day, that which is northerly, braces the body, giving it tone, agility, and color, improves the sense of hearing, dries up the bowels, pinches the eyes, and aggravates any previous pain which may have been seated in the chest. But the southerly relaxes the body, and renders it humid, brings on dullness of hearing, heaviness of the head, and vertigo, impairs the movements of the eyes and the whole body, and renders the alvine discharges watery.

18. With regard to the seasons, in spring and in the commencement of summer, children and those next to them in age are most comfortable, and enjoy best health; in summer and during a certain portion of autumn, old people; during the remainder of the autumn and in winter, those of the intermediate ages.

19. All diseases occur at all seasons of the year, but certain of them are more apt to occur and be exacerbated at certain seasons.

20. The diseases of spring are, maniacal, melancholic, and epileptic disorders, bloody flux, quinsy, coryza, hoarseness, cough, leprosy, lichen alphos, exanthemata mostly ending in ulcerations, tubercles, and arthritic diseases.

21. Of summer, certain of these, and continued, ardent, and tertian fevers, most especially vomiting, diarrhoea, ophthalmy, pains of the ears, ulcerations of the mouth, mortifications of the privy parts, and the sudamina.

22. Of autumn, most of the summer, quartan, and irregular fevers, enlarged spleen, dropsy, phthisis, strangury, lientery, dysentery, sciatica, quinsy, asthma, ileus, epilepsy, maniacal and melancholic disorders.

23. Of winter, pleurisy, pneumonia, coryza, hoarseness, cough, pains of the chest, pains of the ribs and loins, headache, vertigo, and apoplexy.

24. In the different ages the following complaints occur: to little and new-born children, aphthae, vomiting, coughs, sleeplessness, frights, inflammation of the navel, watery discharges from the ears.

25. At the approach of dentition, pruritus of the gums, fevers, convulsions, diarrhoea, especially when cutting the canine teeth, and in those who are particularly fat, and have constipated bowels.

26. To persons somewhat older, affections of the tonsils, incurvation of the spine at the vertebra next the occiput, asthma, calculus, round worms, ascarides, acrochordon, satyriasmus, struma, and other tubercles (phymata), but especially the aforesaid.

27. To persons of a more advanced age, and now on the verge of manhood, the most of these diseases, and, moreover, more chronic fevers, and epistaxis.

28. Young people for the most part have a crisis in their complaints, some in forty days, some in seven months, some in seven years, some at the approach to puberty; and such complaints of children as remain, and do not pass away about puberty, or in females about the commencement of menstruation, usually become chronic.

29. To persons past boyhood, haemoptysis, phthisis, acute fevers, epilepsy, and other diseases, but especially the aforementioned.

30. To persons beyond that age, asthma, pleurisy, pneumonia, lethargy, phrenitis, ardent fevers, chronic diarrhoea, cholera, dysentery, lientery, hemorrhoids.

31. To old people dyspnoea, catarrhs accompanied with coughs, dysuria, pains of the joints, nephritis, vertigo, apoplexy, cachexia, pruritus of the whole body, insomnolency, defluxions of the bowels, of the eyes, and of the nose, dimness of sight, cataract (glaucoma), and dullness of hearing.

SECTION IV.

1. We must purge pregnant women, if matters be turgid (in a state of orgasm?), from the fourth to the seventh month, but less freely in the latter; in the first and last stages of pregnancy it should be avoided.

2. In purging we should bring away such matters from the body as it would be advantageous had they come away spontaneously; but those of an opposite character should be stopped.

3. If the matters which are purged be such as should be purged, it is beneficial and well borne; but if the contrary, with difficulty.

4. We should rather purge upward in summer, and downward in winter.

5. About the time of the dog-days, and before it, the administration of purgatives is unsuitable.

6. Lean persons who are easily made to vomit should be purged upward, avoiding the winter season.

7. Persons who are difficult to vomit, and are moderately fat, should be purged downward, avoiding the summer season.

8. We must be guarded in purging phthisical persons upward.

9. And from the same mode of reasoning, applying the opposite rule to melancholic persons, we must purge them freely downward.

10. In very acute diseases, if matters be in a state of orgasm, we may purge on the first day, for it is a bad thing to procrastinate in such cases.

11. Those cases in which there are tormina, pains about the umbilicus, and pains about the loins, not removed either by purgative medicines or otherwise, usually terminate in dry dropsy.

12. It is a bad thing to purge upward in winter persons whose bowels are in a state of lientery.

13. Persons who are not easily purged upward by the hellebores, should have their bodies moistened by plenty of food and rest before taking the draught.

14. When one takes a draught of hellebore, one should be made to move more about, and indulge less in sleep and repose. Sailing on the sea shows that motion disorders the body.

15. When you wish the hellebore to act more, move the body, and when to stop, let the patient get sleep and rest.

16. Hellebore is dangerous to persons whose flesh is sound, for it induces convulsion.

17. Anorexia, heartburn, vertigo, and a bitter taste of the mouth, in a person free from fever, indicate the want of purging upward.

18. Pains seated above the diaphragm indicate purging upward, and those below it, downward.

19. Persons who have no thirst while under the action of a purgative medicine, do not cease from being purged until they become thirsty.

20. If persons free from fever be seized with tormina, heaviness of the knees, and pains of the loins, this indicates that purging downward is required.

21. Alvine dejections which are black, like blood, taking place spontaneously, either with or without fever, are very bad; and the more numerous and unfavorable the colors, so much the worse; when with medicine it is better, and a variety of colors in this case is not bad.

22. When black bile is evacuated in the beginning of any disease whatever, either upward or downward, it is a mortal symptom.

23. In persons attenuated from any disease, whether acute or chronic, or from wounds, or any other cause, if there be a discharge either of black bile, or resembling black blood, they die on the following day.

24. Dysentery, if it commence with black bile, is mortal.

25. Blood discharged upward, whatever be its character, is a bad symptom, but downward it is (more?) favorable, and so also black dejections.

26. If in a person ill of dysentery, substances resembling flesh be discharged from the bowels, it is a mortal symptom.

27. In whatever cases of fever there is a copious hemorrhage from whatever channel, the bowels are in a loose state during convalescence.

28. In all cases whatever, bilious discharges cease if deafness supervenes, and in all cases deafness ceases when bilious discharges supervene.

29. Rigors which occur on the sixth day have a difficult crisis.

30. Diseases attended with paroxysms, if at the same hour that the fever leaves it return again next day, are of difficult crisis.

31. In febrile diseases attended with a sense of lassitude, deposits form about the joints, and especially those of the jaws.

32. In convalescents from diseases, if any part be pained, there deposits are formed.

33. But if any part be in a painful state previous to the illness, there the disease fixes.

34. If a person laboring under a fever, without any swelling in the fauces, be seized with a sense of suffocation suddenly, it is a mortal symptom.

35. If in a person with fever, the become suddenly distorted, and he cannot swallow unless with difficulty, although no swelling be present, it is a mortal symptom.

36. Sweats, in febrile diseases, are favorable, if they set in on the third, fifth, seventh, ninth, eleventh, fourteenth, seventeenth, twenty-first, twenty-seventh, and thirty-fourth day, for these sweats prove a crisis to the disease; but sweats not occurring thus, indicate pain, a protracted disease, and relapses.

37. Cold sweats occurring with an acute fever, indicate death; and along with a milder one, a protracted disease.

38. And in whatever part of the body there is a sweat, it shows that the disease is seated there.

39. And in whatever part of the body heat or cold is seated, there is disease.

40. And wherever there are changes in the whole body, and if the body be alternately cold and hot, or if one color succeed another, this indicates a protracted disease.

41. A copious sweat after sleep occuring without any manifest cause, indicates that the body is using too much food. But if it occur when one is not taking food, it indicates that evacuation is required.

42. A copious sweat, whether hot or cold, flowing continuously, indicates, the cold a greater, and the hot a lesser disease.

43. Fevers, not of the intermittent type, which are exacerbated on the third day, are dangerous; but if they intermit in any form, this indicates that they are not dangerous.

44. In cases attended with protracted fevers, tubercles (phymata) or pains occur about the joints.

45. When tubercles (phymata) or pains attack the joints after fevers, such persons are using too much food.

46. If in a fever not of the intermittent type a rigor seize a person already much debilitated, it is mortal.

47. In fevers not of the intermittent type, expectorations which are livid bloody, fetid and bilious, are all bad; but if evacuated properly, they are favorable. So it is with the alvine evacuations and the urine. But if none of the proper excretions take place by these channels, it is bad.

48. In fevers not of the intermittent type, if the external parts be cold, but the internal be burnt up, and if there be thirst, it is a mortal symptom.

49. In a fever not of the intermittent type, if a lip, an eyebrow, an eye, or the nose, be distorted; or if there be loss of sight or of hearing, and the patient be in a weak state—whatever of these symptoms occur, death is at hand.

50. Apostemes in fevers which are not resolved at the first crisis, indicate a protracted disease.

51. When in a fever not of the intermittent type dyspnoea and delirium come on, the case is mortal.

52. When persons in fevers, or in other illnesses, shed tears voluntarily, it is nothing out of place; but when they shed tears involuntarily, it is more so.

53. In whatever cases of fever very viscid concretions form about the teeth, the fevers turn out to be particularly strong.

54. In whatever case of ardent fever dry coughs of a tickling nature with slight expectoration are long protracted, there is usually not much thirst.

55. All fevers complicated with buboes are bad, except ephemerals.

56. Sweat supervening in a case of the fever ceasing, is bad, for the disease is protracted, and it indicates more copious humors.

57. Fever supervening in a case of confirmed spasm, or of tetanus, removes the disease.

58. A rigor supervening in a case of ardent fever, produces resolution of it.

59. A true tertian comes to a crisis in seven periods at furthest.

60. When in fevers there is deafness, if blood run from the nostrils, or the bowels become disordered, it carries off the disease.

61. In a febrile complaint, if the fever do not leave on the odd days, it relapses.

62. When jaundice supervenes in fevers before the seventh day, it a bad symptom, unless there be watery discharges from the bowels.

63. In whatever cases of fever rigors occur during the day, the fevers come to a resolution during the day.

64. When in cases of fever jaundice occurs on the seventh, the ninth, the eleventh, or the fourteenth day, it is a good symptom, provided the hypochondriac region be not hard. Otherwise it is not a good symptom.

65. A strong heat about the stomach and cardialgia are bad symptoms in fevers.

66. In acute fevers, spasms, and strong pains about the bowels are bad symptoms.

67. In fevers, frights after sleep, or convulsions, are a bad symptom.

68. In fevers, a stoppage of the respiration is a bad symptom, for it indicates convulsions.

69. When the urine is thick, grumoss, and scanty in cases not free from fever a copious discharge of thinner urine proves beneficial. Such a discharge more commonly takes place when the urine has had a sediment from the first, or soon after the commencement.

70. When in fevers the urine is turbid, like that of a beast of burden, in such a case there either is or will be headache.

71. In cases which come to a crisis on the seventh day, the urine has a red nubecula on the fourth day, and the other symptoms accordingly.

72. When the urine is transparent and white, it is bad; it appears principally in cases of phrenitis.

73. When the hypochondriac region is affected with meteorism and borborygmi, should pain of the loins supervene, the bowels get into a loose and watery state, unless there be an eruption of flatus or a copious evacuation of urine. These things occur in fevers.

74. When there is reason to expect that an abscess will form in joints, the abscess is carried off by a copious discharge of urine, which is thick, and becomes white, like what begins to form in certain cases of quartan fever, attended with a sense of lassitude. It is also speedily carried off by a hemorrhage from the nose.

75. Blood or pus in the urine indicates ulceration either of the kidneys or of the bladder.

76. When small fleshy substances like hairs are discharged along with thick urine, these substances come from the kidneys.

77. In those cases where there are furfuraceous particles discharged along with thick urine, there is scabies of the bladder.

78. In those cases where there is a spontaneous discharge of bloody urine, it indicates rupture of a small vein in the kidneys.

79. In those cases where there is a sandy sediment in the urine, there is calculus in the bladder (or kidneys).

80. If a patient pass blood and clots in his urine, and have strangury, and if a pain seize the hypogastric region and perineum, the parts about the bladder are affected.

81. If a patient pass blood, pus, and scales, in the urine, and if it have a heavy smell, ulceration of the bladder is indicated.

82. When tubercles form in the urethra, if these suppurate and burst, there is relief.

83. When much urine is passed during the night, it indicates that the alvine evacuations are scanty.

SECTION V.

1. A spasm from taking hellebore is of a fatal nature.

2. Spasm supervening on a wound is fatal.

3. A convulsion, or hiccup, supervening on a copious discharge of blood is bad.

4. A convulsion, or hiccup, supervening upon hypercatharsis is bad.

5. If a drunken person suddenly lose his speech, he will die convulsed, unless fever come on, or he recover his speech at the time when the consequences of a debauch pass off.

6. Such persons as are seized with tetanus die within four days, or if they pass these they recover.

7. Those cases of epilepsy which come on before puberty may undergo a change; but those which come on after twenty-five years of age, for the most part terminate in death.

8. In pleuritic affections, when the disease is not purged off in fourteen days, it usually terminates in empyema.

9. Phthisis most commonly occurs between the ages of eighteen and thirty-five years.

10. Persons who escape an attack of quinsy, and when the disease is turned upon the lungs, die in seven days; or if they pass these they become affected with empyema.

11. In persons affected with phthisis, if the sputa which they cough up have a heavy smell when poured upon coals, and if the hairs of the head fall off, the case will prove fatal.

12. Phthisical persons, the hairs of whose head fall off, die if diarrhoea set in.

13. In persons who cough up frothy blood, the discharge of it comes from the lungs.

14. Diarrhoea attacking a person affected with phthisis is a mortal symptom.

15. Persons who become affected with empyema after pleurisy, if they get clear of it in forty days from the breaking of it, escape the disease; but if not, it passes into phthisis.

16. Heat produces the following bad effects on those who use it frequently: enervation of the fleshy parts, impotence of the nerves, torpor of the understanding, hemorrhages, deliquia, and, along with these, death.

17. Cold induces convulsions, tetanus, mortification, and febrile rigors.

18. Cold is inimical to the bones, the teeth, the nerves, the brain, and the spinal marrow, but heat is beneficial.

19. Such parts as have been congealed should be heated, except where there either is a hemorrhage, or one is expected.

20. Cold pinches ulcers, hardens the skin, occasions pain which does not end in suppuration, blackens, produces febrile rigors, convulsions, and tetanus.

21. In the case of a muscular youth having tetanus without a wound, during the midst of summer, it sometimes happens that the allusion of a large quantity of cold water recalls the heat. Heat relieves these diseases.

22. Heat is suppurative, but not in all kinds of sores, but when it is, it furnishes the greatest test of their being free from danger. It softens the skin, makes it thin, removes pain, soothes rigor, convulsions, and tetanus. It removes affections of the head, and heaviness of it. It is particularly efficacious in fractures of the bones, especially of those which have been exposed, and most especially in wounds of the head, and in mortifications and ulcers from cold; in herpes exedens, of the anus, the privy parts, the womb, the bladder, in all these cases heat is agreeable, and brings matters to a crisis; but cold is prejudicial, and does mischief.

23. Cold water is to be applied in the following cases; when there is a hemorrhage, or when it is expected, but not applied to the spot, but around the spot whence the blood flows; and in inflammations and inflammatory affections, inclining to a red and subsaguineous color, and consisting of fresh blood, in these cases it is to be applied but it occasions mortification in old cases; and in erysipelas not attended with ulceration, as it proves injurious to erysipelas when ulcerated.

24. Cold things, such as snow and ice, are inimical to the chest, being provocative of coughs, of discharges of blood, and of catarrhs.

25. Swellings and pains in the joints, ulceration, those of a gouty nature, and sprains, are generally improved by a copious affusion of cold water, which reduces the swelling, and removes the pain; for a moderate degree of numbness removes pain.

26. The lightest water is that which is quickly heated and quickly cooled.

27. When persons have intense thirst, it is a good thing if they can sleep off the desire of drinking.

28. Fumigation with aromatics promotes menstruation, and would be useful in many other cases, if it did not occasion heaviness of the head.

29. Women in a state of pregnancy may be purged, if there be any urgent necessity (or, if the humors be in a state of orgasm?), from the fourth to the seventh month, but less so in the latter case. In the first and last periods it must be avoided.

30. It proves fatal to a woman in a state of pregnancy, if she be seized with any of the acute diseases.

31. If a woman with child be bled, she will have an abortion, and this will be the more likely to happen, the larger the foetus.

32. Haemoptysis in a woman is removed by an eruption of the menses.

33. In a woman when there is a stoppage the menses, a discharge of blood from the nose is good.

34. When a pregnant woman has a violent diarrhoea, there is danger of her miscarrying.

35. Sneezing occurring to a woman affected with hysterics, and in difficult labor, is a good symptom.

36. When the menstrual discharge is of a bad color and irregular, it indicates that the woman stands in need of purging.

37. In a pregnant woman, if the breasts suddenly lose their fullness, she has a miscarriage.

38. If, in a woman pregnant with twins, either of her breasts lose its fullness, she will part with one of her children; and if it be the right breast which becomes slender, it will be the male child, or if the left, the female.

39. If a woman who is not with child, nor has brought forth, have milk, her menses are obstructed.

40. In women, blood collected in the breasts indicates madness.

41. If you wish to ascertain if a woman be with child, give her hydromel to drink when she is going to sleep, and has not taken supper, and if she be seized with tormina in the belly, she is with child, but otherwise she is not pregnant.

42. A woman with child, if it be a male, has a good color, but if a female, she has a bad color.

43. If erysipelas of the womb seize a woman with child, it will probably prove fatal.

44. Women who are very lean, have miscarriages when they prove with child, until they get into better condition.

45. When women, in a moderate condition of body, miscarry in the second or third month, without any obvious cause, their cotyledones are filled with mucosity, and cannot support the weight of the foetus, but are broken asunder.

46. Such women as are immoderately fat, and do not prove with child, in them it is because the epiploon (fat?) blocks up the mouth of the womb, and until it be reduced, they do not conceive.

47. If the portion of the uterus seated near the hip-joint suppurate, it gets into a state requiring to be treated with tents.

48. The male foetus is usually seated in the right, and the female in the left side.

49. To procure the expulsion of the secundines, apply a sternutatory, and shut the nostrils and mouth.

50. If you wish to stop the menses in a woman, apply as large a cupping instrument as possible to the breasts.

51. When women are with child, the mouth of their womb is closed.

52. If in a woman with child, much milk flow from the breasts, it indicates that the foetus is weak; but if the breasts be firm, it indicates that the foetus is in a more healthy state.

53. In women that are about to miscarry, the breasts become slender; but if again they become hard, there will be pain, either in the breasts, or in the hip-joints, or in the eyes, or in the knees, and they will not miscarry.

54. When the mouth of the uterus is hard, it is also necessarily shut.

55. Women with child who are seized with fevers, and who are greatly emaciated, without any (other?) obvious cause, have difficult and dangerous labors, and if they miscarry, they are in danger.

56. In the female flux (immoderate menstruation?), if convulsion and deliquium come on, it is bad.

57. When the menses are excessive, diseases take place, and when the menses are stopped, diseases from the uterus take place.

58. Strangury supervenes upon inflammation of the rectum, and of the womb, and strangury supervenes upon suppuration of the kidney, and hiccup upon inflammation of the liver.

59. If a woman do not conceive, and wish to ascertain whether she can conceive, having wrapped her up in blankets, fumigate below, and if it appear that the scent passes through the body to the nostrils and mouth, know that of herself she is not unfruitful.

60. If woman with a child have her courses, it is impossible that the child can be healthy.

61. If a woman's courses be suppressed, and neither rigor nor fever has followed, but she has been affected with nausea, you may reckon her to be with child.

62. Women who have the uterus cold and dense (compact?) do not conceive; and those also who have the uterus humid, do not conceive, for the semen is extinguished, and in women whose uterus is very dry, and very hot, the semen is lost from the want of food; but women whose uterus is in an intermediate state between these temperaments prove fertile.

63. And in like manner with respect to males; for either, owing to the laxity of the body, the pneuma is dissipated outwardly, so as not to propel the semen, or, owing to its density, the fluid (semen?) does not pass outwardly; or, owing to coldness, it is not heated so as to collect in its proper place (seminal vessels?), or, owing to its heat, the very same thing happens.

64. It is a bad thing to give milk to persons having headache, and it is also bad to give it in fevers, and to persons whose hypochondria are swelled up, and troubled with borborygmi, and to thirsty persons; it is bad also, when given to those who have bilious discharges in acute fevers, and to those who have copious discharges of blood; but it is suitable in phthisical cases, when not attended with very much fever; it is also to be given in fevers of a chronic and weak nature, when none of the aforementioned symptoms are present, and the patients are excessively emaciated.

65. When swellings appear on wounds, such cases are not likely to be attacked either with convulsions, or delirium, but when these disappear suddenly, if situated behind, spasms and tetanus supervene, and if before, mania, acute pains of the sides, or suppurations, or dysentery, if the swellings be rather red.

66. When no swelling appears on severe and bad wounds, it is a great evil.

67. In such cases, the soft are favorable; and crude, unfavorable.

68. When a person is pained in the back part of the head, he is benefited by having the straight vein in the forehead opened.

69. Rigors commence in women, especially at the loins, and spread by the back to the head; and in men also, rather in the posterior than the anterior side of the body, as from the arms and thighs; the skin there is rare, as is obvious from the growth of hair on them.

70. Persons attacked with quartans are not readily attacked with convulsions, or if previously attacked with convulsions, they cease if a quartan supervene.

71. In those persons in whom the skin is stretched, and parched and hard, the disease terminates without sweats; but in those in whom the skin is loose and rare, it terminates with sweats.

72. Persons disposed to jaundice are not very subject to flatulence.

SECTION VI.

1. In cases of chronic lientery, acid eructations supervening when there were none previously, is a good symptom.

2. Persons whose noses are naturally watery, and their seed watery, have rather a deranged state of health; but those in the opposite state, a more favorable.

3. In protracted cases of dysentery, loathing of food is a bad symptom, and still worse, if along with fever.

4. Ulcers, attended with a falling off of the hair, are mali moris.

5. It deserves to be considered whether the pains in the sides, and in the breasts, and in the other parts, differ much from one another.

6. Diseases about the kidneys and bladder are cured with difficulty in old men.

7. Pains occurring about the stomach, the more superficial they are, the more slight are they; and the less superficial, the more severe.

8. In dropsical persons, ulcers forming on the body are not easily healed.

9. Broad exanthemata are not very itchy.

10. In a person having a painful spot in the head, with intense cephalalgia, pus or water running from the nose, or by the mouth, or at the ears, removes the disease.

11. Hemorrhoids appearing in melancholic and nephritic affections are favorable.

12. When a person has been cured of chronic hemorrhoids, unless one be left, there is danger of dropsy or phthisis supervening.

13. Sneezing coming on, in the case of a person afflicted with hiccup, removes the hiccup.

14. In a case of dropsy, when the water runs by the veins into the belly, it removes the disease.

15. In confirmed diarrhoea, vomiting, when it comes on spontaneously, removes the diarrhoea.

16. A diarrhoea supervening in a confirmed case of pleurisy or pneumonia is bad.

17. It is a good thing in ophthalmy for the patient to be seized with diarrhoea.

18. A severe wound of the bladder, of the brain, of the heart, of the diaphragm, of the small intestines, of the stomach, and of the liver, is deadly.

19. When a bone, cartilage, nerve, the slender part of the jaw, or prepuce, are cut out, the part is neither restored, nor does it unite.

20. If blood be poured out preternaturally into a cavity, it must necessarily become corrupted.

21. In maniacal affections, if varices or hemorrhoids come on, they remove the mania.

22. Those ruptures in the back which spread down to the elbows are removed by venesection.

23. If a fright or despondency lasts for a long time, it is a melancholic affection.

24. If any of the intestines be transfixed, it does not unite.

25. It is not a good sign for an erysipelas spreading outwardly to be determined inward; but for it to be determined outward from within is good.

26. In whatever cases of ardent fever tremors occur, they are carried off by a delirium.

27. Those cases of empyema or dropsy which are treated by incision or the cautery, if the water or pus flow rapidly all at once, certainly prove fatal.

28. Eunuchs do not take the gout, nor become bald.

29. A woman does not take the gout, unless her menses be stopped.

30. A young man does not take the gout until he indulges in coition.

31. Pains of the eyes are removed by drinking pure wine, or the bath, or a fomentation, or venesection, or purging.

32. Persons whose speech has become impaired are likely to be seized with chronic diarrhoea.

33. Persons having acid eructations are not very apt to be seized with pleurisy.

34. Persons who have become bald are not subject to large varices; but should varices supervene upon persons who are bald, their hair again grows thick.

35. Hiccup supervening in dropsical cases is bad.

36. Venesection cures dysuria; open the internal veins of the arm.

37. It is a good symptom when swelling on the outside of the neck seizes a person very ill of quinsy, for the disease is turned outwardly.

38. It is better not to apply any treatment in cases of occult cancer; for, if treated, the patients die quickly; but if not treated, they hold out for a long time.

39. Convulsions take place either from repletion or depletion; and so it is with hiccup.

40. When pains, without inflammation, occur about the hypochondria, in such cases, fever supervening removes the pain.

41. When pus formed anywhere in the body does not point, this is owing to the thickness of the part.

42. In cases of jaundice, it is a bad symptom when the liver becomes indurated.

43. When persons having large spleens are seized with dysentery, and if the dysentery pass into a chronic state, either dropsy or lientery supervenes, and they die.

44. When ileus comes on in a case of strangury, they prove fatal in seven days, unless, fever supervening, there be a copious discharge of urine.

45. When ulcers continue open for a year or upward, there must necessarily be exfoliation of bone, and the cicatrices are hollow.

46. Such persons as become hump-backed from asthma or cough before puberty, die.

47. Persons who are benefited by venesection or purging, should be bled or purged in spring.

48. In enlargement of the spleen, it is a good symptom when dysentery comes on.

49. In gouty affections, the inflammation subsides in the course of forty days.

50. When the brain is severely wounded, fever and vomiting of bile necessarily supervene.

51. When persons in good health are suddenly seized with pains in the head, and straightway are laid down speechless, and breathe with stertor, they die in seven days, unless fever come on.

52. We must attend to the appearances of the eyes in sleep, as presented from below; for if a portion of the white be seen between the closed eyelids, and if this be not connected with diarrhaea or severe purging, it is a very bad and mortal symptom.

53. Delirium attended with laughter is less dangerous than delirium attended with a serious mood.

54. In acute diseases, complicated with fever, a moaning respiration is bad.

55. For the most part, gouty affections rankle in spring and in autumn.

56. In melancholic affections, determinations of the humor which occasions them produce the following diseases; either apoplexy of the whole body, or convulsion, or madness, or blindness.

57. Persons are most subject to apoplexy between the ages of forty and sixty.

58. If the omentum protrude, it necessarily mortifies and drops off.

59. In chronic diseases of the hip-joint, if the bone protrude and return again into its socket, there is mucosity in the place.

60. In persons affected with chronic disease of the hip-joint, if the bone protrude from its socket, the limb becomes wasted and maimed, unless the part be cauterized.

SECTION VII.

1. In acute diseases, coldness of the extremities is bad.

2. Livid flesh on a diseased bone is bad.

3. Hiccup and redness of the eyes, when they supervene on vomiting, are bad.

4. A chill supervening on a sweat is not good.

5. Dysentery, or dropsy, or ecstacy coming on madness is good.

6. In a very protracted disease, loss of appetite and unmixed discharges from the bowels are bad symptoms.

7. A rigor and delirium from excessive drinking are bad.

8. From the rupture of an internal abscess, prostration of strength, vomiting, and deliquium animi result.

9. Delirium or convulsion from a flow of blood is bad.

10. Vomiting, or hiccup, or convulsion, or delirium, in ileus, is bad.

11. Pneumonia coming on pleurisy is bad.

12. Phrenitis along with pneumonia is bad.

13. Convulsion or tetanus, coming upon severe burning, is bad.

14. Stupor or delirium from a blow on the head is bad.

15. From a spitting of blood there is a spitting of pus.

16. From spitting of pus arise phthisis and a flux; and when the sputa are stopped, they die.

17. Hiccup in inflammation of the liver is bad.

18. Convulsion or delirium supervening upon insomnolency is bad.

18a. Trembling upon lethargus is bad.

19. Erysipelas upon exposure of a bone (is bad?).

20. Mortification or suppuration upon erysipelas is bad.

21. Hemorrhage upon a strong pulsation in wounds is bad.

22. Suppuration upon a protracted pain of the parts about the bowels is bad.

23. Dysentery upon unmixed alvine discharges is bad.

24. Delirium upon division of the cranium, if it penetrate into the cavity of the head, is bad.

25. Convulsion upon severe purging is mortal.

26. Upon severe pain of the parts about the bowels, coldness of the extremities coming on is bad.

27. Tenesmus coming on in a case of pregnancy causes abortion.

28. Whatever piece of bone, cartilage, or nerve (tendon?) is cut off, it neither grows nor unites.

29. When strong diarrhoea supervenes in a case of leucophlegmatia, it removes the disease.

30. In those cases in which frothy discharges occur in diarrhoea there are defluxions from the head.

31. When there is a farinaceous sediment in the urine during fever, it indicates a protracted illness.

32. In those cases in which the urine is thin at first, and the sediments become bilious, an acute disease is indicated.

33. In those cases in which the urine becomes divided there is great disorder in the body.

34. When bubbles settle on the surface of the urine, they indicate disease of the kidneys, and that the complaint will be protracted.

35. When the scum on the surface is fatty and copious, it indicates acute diseases of the kidneys.

36. Whenever the aforementioned symptoms occur in nephritic diseases, and along with them acute pains about the muscles of the back, provided these be seated about the external parts, you may expect that there will be an abscess; but if the pains be rather about the internal parts, you may also rather expect that the abscess will be seated internally.

37. Haematemesis, without fever, does not prove fatal, but with fever it is bad; it is to be treated with refrigerant and styptic things.

38. Defluxions into the cavity of the chest suppurate in twenty days.

39. When a patient passes blood and clots, and is seized with strangury and pain in the perineum and pubes, disease about the bladder is indicated.

40. If the tongue suddenly lose its powers, or a part of the body become apoplectic, the affection is of a melancholic nature.

41. In hypercatharsis, of old persons, hiccup supervening is not a good symptom.

42. In a fever, is not of a bilious nature, a copious allusion of hot water upon the head removes the fever.

43. A woman does not become ambidexterous.

44. When empyema is treated either by the cautery or incision, if pure and white pus flow from the wound, the patients recover; but if mixed with blood, slimy and fetid, they die.

45. When abscess of the liver is treated by the cautery or incision, if the pus which is discharged be pure and white, the patients recover, (for in this case it is situated in the coats of the liver;) but if it resemble the lees of oil as it flows, they die.

46. Pains of the eyes are removed by drinking undiluted wine, plenteous bathing with hot water, and venesection.

47. If a dropsical patient be seized with hiccup the case is hopeless.

48. Strangury and dysuria are cured by drinking pure wine, and venesection; open the vein on the inside.

49. It is a good sign when swelling and redness on the breast seize a person very ill of quinsy, for in this case the disease is diverted outwardly.

50. When the brain is attacked with sphacelus, the patients die in three days; or if they escape these, they recover.

51. Sneezing arises from the head, owing to the brain being heated, or the cavity (ventricle) in the head being filled with humors; the air confined in it then is discharged, and makes a noise, because it comes through a narrow passage.

52. Fever supervening on painful affections of the liver removes the pain.

53. Those persons to whom it is beneficial to have blood taken from their veins, should have it done in spring.

54. In those cases where phlegm is collected between the diaphragm and the stomach, and occasions pain, as not finding a passage into either of the cavities, the disease will be carried off if the phlegm be diverted to the bladder by the veins.

55. When the liver is filled with water and bursts into the epiploon, in this case the belly is filled with water and the patient dies.

56. Anxiety, yawning, rigor,—wine drunk with an equal proportion of water, removes these complaints.

57. When tubercles (phymata) form in the urethra, if they suppurate and burst, the pain is carried off.

58. In cases of concussion of the brain produced by any cause, the patients necessarily lose their speech.

59. In a person affected with fever, when there is no swelling in the fauces, should suffocation suddenly come on, and the patient not be able to swallow, except with difficulty, it is a mortal symptom.

59a. In the case of a person oppressed by fever, if the neck be turned aside, and the patient cannot swallow, while there is no swelling in the neck, it is a mortal sign.

60. Fasting should be prescribed to the those persons who have humid flesh; for fasting dries bodies.

61. When there are changes in the whole body, and the body becomes sometimes cold and sometimes hot, and the color changes, a protracted disease is indicated.

62. A copious sweat, hot or cold, constantly flowing, indicates a superabundance of humidity; we must evacuate then, in a strong person upward, and in a weak, downward.

63. Fevers, not of the intermittent type, if they become exacerbated every third day are dangerous; but if they intermit in any form whatever, this shows that they are not dangerous.

64. In cases of protracted fever, either chronic abscesses or pains in the joints come on.

65. When chronic abscesses (phymata) or pains in the joints take place after fevers, the patients are using too much food.

66. If one give to a person in fever the same food which is given to a person in good health, what is strength to the one is disease to the other.

67. We must look to the urinary evacuations, whether they resemble those of persons in health; if not at all so, they are particularly morbid, but if they are like those of healthy persons, they are not at all morbid.

68. When the dejections are allowed to stand and not shaken, and a sediment is formed like scrapings (of the bowels), in such a case it is proper to purge the bowels; and if you give ptisans before purging, the more you give the more harm you will do.

69. Crude dejections are the product of black bile; if abundant, of more copious, and if deficient, of less copious collections of it.

70. The sputa in fevers, not of an intermittent type, which are livid, streaked with blood, and fetid, are all bad, it is favorable when this evacuation, like the urinary and alvine, passes freely; and whenever any discharge is suppressed and not purged off it is bad.

71. When you wish to purge the body, you must bring it into a state favorable to evacuations; and if you wish to dispose it to evacuations upward, you must bind the belly; and if you wish to dispose it to evacuations downward, you must moisten the belly.

72. Sleep and watchfulness, both of them, when immoderate, constitute disease.

73. In fevers which do not intermit, if the external parts be cold, and the internal burning hot, and fever prevail, it is a mortal sign.

74. In a fever which does not intermit, if a lip, the nose, or an eye be distorted, if the patient lose his sense of sight or of hearing, while now in a weak state,—whatever of these symptoms occurs it is mortal.

75. Upon leucophlegmatia dropsy supervenes.

76. Upon diarrhoea dysentery.

77. Upon dysentery lientery.

78. Upon sphacelus exfoliation of the bone.

79 and 80. Upon vomiting of blood consumption, and a purging of pus upward; upon consumption a defluxion from the head; upon a defluxion diarrhoea; upon diarrhoea a stoppage of the purging upward; upon the stoppage of it death.

81. In the discharges by the bladder, the belly, and the flesh (the skin?) if the body has departed slightly from its natural condition, the disease is slight; if much, it is great; if very much, it is mortal.

82. Persons above forty years of age who are affected with frenzy, do not readily recover; the danger is less when the disease is cognate to the constitution and age.

83. In whatever diseases the eyes weep voluntarily, it is a good symptom, but when involuntarily, it is a bad.

84. When in quartan fevers blood flows from the nostrils it is a bad symptom.

85. Sweats are dangerous when they do not occur on critical days, when they are strong, and quickly forced out of the forehead, either in the form of drops or in streams, and if excessively cold and copious; for such a sweat must proceed from violence, excess of pain, and prolonged squeezing (affliction?).

86. In a chronic disease an excessive flux from the bowels is bad.

87. Those diseases which medicines do not cure, iron (the knife?) cures; those which iron cannot cure, fire cures; and those which fire cannot cure, are to be reckoned wholly incurable.

ON THE SURGERY

IT IS the business of the physician to know, in the first place, things similar and things dissimilar; those connected with things most important, most easily known, and in anywise known; which are to be seen, touched, and heard; which are to be perceived in the sight, and the touch, and the hearing, and the nose, and the tongue, and the understanding; which are to be known by all the means we know other things.

2. The things relating to surgery, are—the patient; the operator; the assistants; the instruments; the light, where and how; how many things, and how; where the body, and the instruments; the time; the manner; the place.

3. The operator is either sitting or standing, conveniently for himself, for the person operated upon, for the light. There are two kinds of light, the common and the artificial; the common is not at our disposal, the artificial is at our disposal. There are two modes of using each, either to the light, or from the light (to the side?). There is little use of that which is from (or oblique to the light), and the degree of it is obvious. As to opposite the light, we must turn the part to be operated upon to that which is most brilliant of present and convenient lights, unless those parts which should be concealed, and which it is a shame to look upon; thus the part that is operated upon should be opposite the light, and the operator opposite the part operated upon, except in so far as he does not stand in his own light; for in this case the operator will indeed see, but the thing operated upon will

not be seen. With regard to himself when sitting, his feet should be raised to a direct line with his knees, and nearly in contact with one another; the knees a little higher than the groins, and at some distance from one another, for the elbows to rest upon them. The robe, in a neat and orderly manner, is to be thrown over the elbows and shoulders equally and proportionally. With regard to the part operated upon; we have to consider how far distant, and how near, above, below, on this side on that side, or in the middle. The measure as to distance and proximity is, that the elbows do not press the knees before, nor the sides behind; that the hands be not raised higher than the breasts, nor lower than so as that when the breast reposes on the knees he may have the hands at right angles with the arm: thus it is as regards the medium; but as concerns this side or that, the operator must not be beyond his be beyond his seat, but in proportion as he may require turning he must shift the body, or part of the body, that is operated upon. When standing, he must make his inspection, resting firmly and equally on both feet; but he must operate while supporting himself upon either leg, and not the one on the same side with the hand which he makes use of; the knee being raised to the height of the groins as while sitting; and the other measures in like manner. The person operated upon should accommodate the operator with regard to the other parts of his body, either standing, sitting, or lying; so as that he may continue to preserve his figure, avoid sinking down, shrinking from, turning away; and may maintain the figure and position of the part operated upon, during the act of presentation, during the operation, and in the subsequent position.

4. The nails should be neither longer nor shorter than the points of the fingers; and the surgeon should practice with the extremities of the fingers, the index-finger being usually turned to the thumb; when using the entire hand, it should be prone; when both hands, they should be opposed to one another. It greatly promotes a dexterous use of the fingers when the space between them is large, and when the thumb is opposed to the index. But it is clearly a disease when the thumb is impaired from birth, or when, from a habit contracted during the time of nursing, it is impeded in its motions by the fingers. One should practice all sorts of work with either of with either of them, and with both together (for they are both alike), endeavouring to do them well, elegantly, quickly, without trouble, neatly, and promptly.

5. The instruments, and when and how they should be prepared, will be treated of afterwards; so that they may not impede the work, and that there may be no difficulty in taking hold of them, with the part of the body which operates. But if another gives them, he must be ready a little beforehand, and do as you direct.

6. Those about the patient must present the part to be operated upon as may seem proper, and they must hold the rest of the body steady, in silence, and listening to the commands of the operator.

7. There are two views of bandaging: that which regards it while doing, and that which regards it when done. It should be done quickly, by despatching the without pain, by being readily done; with ease, by being prepared for everything; and with elegance, so that it may be agreeable to the sight. By what mode of training these accomplishments are to be acquired has been stated. When done, it should fit well and neatly; it is neatly done when with judgment, and when it is equal and unequal, according as the parts are equal or unequal. The forms of it (the bandage?) are the simple, the slightly winding (called ascia), the sloping (sima), the monoculus, the rhombus, and the semirhombus. The form of bandage should be suitable to the form and the affection of the part to which it is applied.

8. There are two useful purposes to be fulfilled by bandaging: (first,) strength, which is imparted by the compression and the number of folds. In one case the bandage effects the cure, and in another it contributes to the cure. For these purposes this is the rule—that the force of the constriction be such as to prevent the adjoining parts from separating, without compressing them much, and so that the parts may be adjusted but not forced together; and that the constriction be small at the extremities, and least of all in the middle. The knot and the thread that is passed through should not be in a downward but in an upward direction, regard being had to the circumstances under which the case is presented; to position, to the bandaging, and to the compression. The commencement of the ligatures is not to be placed at the wound, but where the kriot is situated. The knot should not be placed where it will be exposed to friction, nor where it will be in the way, nor where it will be useless. The knot and the thread should be soft, and not large.

9. (Second.) One ought to be well aware that every bandage has a tendency to fall off towards the part that declines or becomes smaller; as, for example, upwards, in the case of the head, and downwards, in the case of the leg. The turns of the bandage should be made from right to left, and from left to right, except on the head, where it should be in a straight direction. When opposite parts are to be bandaged together, we must use a bandage with two heads; or if we make use of a bandage with one head, we must attach it in like manner at some fixed point: such, for example, as the middle of the head; and so in other cases. Those parts which are much exposed to motion, such as the joints, where there is a flexion, should have few and slight bandages applied to them, as at the ham; but where there is much extension, the bandage should be single and broad, as at the kneepan; and for the maintenance of the bandage in its proper place, some turns should be carried to those parts which are not much moved, and are lank, such as the parts above and below the knee. In the case of the shoulder; a fold should be carried round by the other armpit; in that of the groin, by the flanks of the opposite side; and of the leg, to above the calf of the leg. When the bandage has a tendency to escape above, it should be secured below, and vice versa; and where there is no means of doing this, as in the case of the head, the turns are to be made mostly on the most level part of the head, and the folds are to be done with as little obliquity as possible, so that the firmest part being last applied may secure the portions which are more movable. When we cannot secure the bandaging by means of folds of the cloth, nor by suspending them from the opposite side, we must have recourse to stitching it with ligatures, either passed circularly or in the form of a seam.

10. The bandages should be clean, light, soft, and thin. One should practice rolling with both hands together, and with either separately. One should also choose a suitable one, according to the breadth and thickness of the parts. The heads of the bandages should be hard, smooth, and neatly put on. That sort of bandaging is the worst which quickly falls off; but those are bad bandages which neither compress nor yet come off.

11. The following are the object which the upper bandage, the under bandage, or both aim at: The object of the under bandage is either to bring together parts that are separated, or to compress such as are expanded, or to separate what are contracted, or to restore to shape what are distorted, or the contrary. It is necessary to prepare pieces of linen cloth, which are light, thin, soft, clean, having no seams nor protuberances on them, but sound, and able to bear some stretching, or even a little more than required; not dry, but wetted with a juice suitable to the purpose required. We must deal with parts separated (in a sinus?) in such wise, that the parts which are raised may touch the bottom without producing pressure; we must begin on the sound part, and terminate at the wound; so that whatever humor is in it may be expelled, and that it may be prevented from collecting more. And straight parts are to be bandaged in a straight direction, and oblique obliquely, in such a position as to create no pain; and so that there may be no constriction nor falling off on a change of position, either for the purpose of taking hold of anything, or laying the limb; and that muscles, veins, nerves, and bones may be properly placed and adjusted to one another. It should be raised or laid in a natural position, so as not to occasion pain. In those cases in which an abscess is formed, we must act in a contrary way. When our object is to bring together parts which have become expanded, in other respects we must proceed on the same plain; and we must commence the bringing together from some considerable distance; and after their approach, we must apply compression, at first slight, and afterwards stronger, the limit of it being the actual contact of the parts. In order to separate parts which are drawn together, when attended with inflammation, we must proceed on the opposite plan; but when without inflammation, we must use the same preparations, but bandage in the opposite direction. In order to rectify distorted parts, we must proceed otherwise on the same principles; but the parts which are separated must be brought together by an underbandage, by agglutinants, and by suspending it (the limb?) in its natural position. And when the deformities are the contrary, this is to be done on the contrary plan.

12. In fractures we must attend to the length, breadth, thickness, and number of the compresses. The length should be that of the bandaging; the breadth, three or four fingers; thickness, three or fourfold; number so as to encircle the limb, neither more nor less; those applied for the purpose of rectifying a deformity, should be of such a length as to encircle it; the breadth and thickness being determined by the vacuity, which is not to be filled up at once. The upper bandages are two, the first of which is to be carried from the seat of the injury upwards, and the second from the seat of the injury downwards, and from below upwards; the parts about the seat of the injury being most compressed, the extremities least, and the rest in proportion. The upper bandages should take in a considerable portion of the sound parts. We must attend to the number, length, and breadth of the bandages; the number must be such as not to be inferior to what the injury requires, nor occasion compression with the splints, nor prove cumbersome, nor occasion any slipping of them, nor render them inefficient. As to length and breadth, they should be three, four, five, or six cubits in length, and as many fingers broad. The folds of the strings (selvages?) should be such as not to occasion pressure; they are to be soft and not thick; and all these things are to be proportionate to the length, breadth, and thickness of the part affected. The splints are to be smooth, even, and rounded at the extremities; somewhat less all along than the upper bandaging, and thickest at the part to which fracture inclines. Those parts where there are tuberosities, and which are devoid of flesh, such as the ankles or fingers, we must guard from the splints which are placed over them, either by position, or by their shortness. They are to be secured by the strings in such a manner as not to occasion pressure at first. A soft, consistent, and clean cerate should be rubbed into the folds of the bandage.

13. As to the temperature and quantity of the water used, its heat should be just such as the hand can bear, and it ought to be known that a large quantity is best for producing relaxation and attenuation, whereas a moderate quantity is best for incarnating and softening. The limit to the affusion is, to stop when the parts become swelled up, and before the swelling subsides; for the parts swell up at first, and fall afterward.

14. The object on which to (the limb?) is laid should be soft, smooth, and sloping upwards toward the protuberant parts of the body, such as the heel or hips, so that there may be no projection, nor bending inwards, nor turning aside. The canal (spout or gutter?) should rather comprehend the whole limb than the half of it, attention being paid to the injury and to whatever else appears to create inconvenience.

15. The presentation of the injured part to the physician, the extension, the arrangement, and so forth, are to be regulated according to nature. What is nature in these operations is to be determined by the accomplishment of the object which we have in view, and for this purpose we must look to the part in the state of rest, in its middle state, and to habit; in regard to the state of rest and relaxation, as in the arm, that it be in a line with the hand; and with regard to the medium between flexion and extension, that the forearm be at right angles to the arm; and with regard to habit, it should be considered that some limbs bear certain positions preferably, as, for example, the thighs extension; for in such attitudes the parts can best bear to be placed for a considerable time without a change of posture. And in the change from the state of distention, the muscles, veins, nerves, and bones, when properly arranged and secured, will preserve their relations to one another while the limb is raised or placed.

16. The extension should be most powerful when the largest and thickest bones, or when both are broken; next when the under-bone, and least of all, when the upper. When immoderate, it is injurious, except in the case of children. The limb should be a little elevated. The model by which we judge if the part be properly set is the sound part of the same name, or the part which is its pair.

17. Friction can relax, brace, incarnate, attenuate: hard braces, soft relaxes, much attenuates, and moderate thickens.

18. The following should be the state of matters on the first application of the bandage. The person to whom it has been applied should say that he feels the compression particularly at the seat of the injury, but very little at the extremities; the parts should be adjusted but not pressed together, and that rather by the number of the bandages than by the force of the constriction; and the tightness should rather be on the increase during the first day and night; but on the next it should be less, and on the third the bandages should be loose. On the next day a soft swelling should be observed in the extremities; and on the third day, when the bandaging is loosed, the swelling should be found diminished in size, and this should be the case every time the bandages are removed. At the second application of the bandage, it should be ascertained whether the dressing has been properly done, and then greater compression should be made, and with more bandages; and on the third, still greater, and still more. On the seventh day from the first dressing, when the bandages are loosed, the limb should be found slender and the bones mobile. We must then have recourse to the splints, provided the limb be free of swelling, pruritus, and ulceration, and allow them to remain until twenty days after the accident; but if any suspicions arise, the bandages must be loosed in the interval. The splints should be tightened every third day.

19. The suspending of a fractured limb in a sling, the disposition of it, and the bandaging, all have for their object to preserve it in position. The principal considerations with regard to the position are the habits and the peculiar nature of each of the limbs: the varieties are shown in running, walking, standing, lying, action, repose.

20. It should be kept in mind that exercise strengthens, and inactivity wastes.

21. Compression should be produced by the number of bandages, rather than by the force of the constriction.

22. In cases of ecchymosis, contusions, sprains, or swellings not attended with inflammations, blood is to be expelled from the wound, in greatest quantity to the upper part, and in smallest to the inferior; neither the arm nor the leg should be placed in a declining position: the head of the bandage should be placed on the wound, and there the greatest pressure should be made; the least at the extremities, and intermediately in the middle; the last fold of the bandage should be at the upper part of the body. As to binding and compression, these objects are to be attained rather by the number of the bandages than the force of the constriction; and moreover, in these cases the bandages should be thin, light, soft, clean, broad, sound, so that they may effect their purpose, even without splints. And we must use affusions.

23. Dislocations, sprains, diastases of bones, violent separation, abruption of the extremities of bones, and distrainings, so as to induce varus or valgus, in these cases we must apply the bandages so as not to compress the part whence the displacement took place, and that we may render them tight at the side to which the displacement was, and give the limb an inclination in the opposite direction, and that in an excessive degree. We employ bandages, compresses, suspension of the limb in a sling, attitude, extension, friction, rectification; and along with these the affusion of much water.

24. In treating parts which are atrophied, we must comprehend a considerable part of the sound limb with the bandage, so that by the influx thereby produced, the wasted part may acquire a supply greater than its loss, and may be thus disposed to growth and restoration of its fleshy parts. It is better also to bandage the parts above, as the thigh in the case of the leg, and also the thigh and leg of the opposite side, so that they may be placed in similar circumstances, and may both equally be deprived of motion; and that the supply of nourishment may be alike curtailed and open to both. The compression should be the effect rather of the number of the bandages than of their tightness. We relax first the part most requiring it, and have recourse to that kind of friction which will promote the growth of flesh, and to affusion. No splints.

25. Those things which are for the purpose of giving support and strength to the part, as to the breast, side, head, and so forth, are used in such cases as the following: for pulsations, that there may be no motion in the part; and in separation at the sutures of the skull, in order to give support; and in order to strengthen the chest and head, in coughs, sneezings, and other movements. In all these cases the same measure of bandaging is to be observed, for where the injury is, there the bandage should compress most, and something soft is to be placed below that suits with the complaint; and we must not apply the bandages tighter than just to stop the pulsations from creating disturbance, and that the

separated parts at the sutures may be brought into contact, they must not be such as absolutely to stop the coughs and sneezings, but so as to give support, and, without occasioning uneasiness, prevent the parts from being shaken.

ON THE
SACRED DISEASE

IT IS THUS with regard to the disease called Sacred: it appears to me to be nowise more divine nor more sacred than other diseases, but has a natural cause from the originates like other affections. Men regard its nature and cause as divine from ignorance and wonder, because it is not at all like to other diseases. And this notion of its divinity is kept up by their inability to comprehend it, and the simplicity of the mode by which it is cured, for men are freed from it by purifications and incantations. But if it is reckoned divine because it is wonderful, instead of one there are many diseases which would be sacred; for, as I will show, there are others no less wonderful and prodigious, which nobody imagines to be sacred. The quotidian, tertian, and quartan fevers, seem to me no less sacred and divine in their origin than this disease, although they are not reckoned so wonderful. And I see men become mad and demented from no manifest cause, and at the same time doing many things out of place; and I have known many persons in sleep groaning and crying out, some in a state of suffocation, some jumping up and fleeing out of doors, and deprived of their reason until they awaken, and afterward becoming well and rational as before, although they be pale and weak; and this will happen not once but frequently. And there are many and various things of the like kind, which it would be tedious to state particularly.

They who first referred this malady to the gods appear to me to have been just such persons as the conjurors, purificators, mountebanks, and charlatans now are, who give themselves out for being excessively religious, and as knowing more than other people. Such persons, then, using the divinity as a pretext and screen of their own inability to of their own inability to afford any assistance, have given out that the disease is sacred, adding suitable reasons for this opinion, they have instituted a mode of treatment which is safe for themselves, namely, by applying purifications and incantations, and enforcing abstinence from baths and many articles of food which are unwholesome to men in diseases. Of sea substances, the surmullet, the blacktail, the mullet, and the eel; for these are the fishes most to be guarded against. And of fleshes, those of the goat, the stag, the sow, and the dog: for these are the kinds of flesh which are aptest to disorder the bowels. Of fowls, the cock, the turtle, and the bustard, and such others as are reckoned to be particularly strong. And of potherbs, mint, garlic, and onions; for what is acrid does not agree with a weak person. And they forbid to have a black robe, because black is expressive of death; and to sleep on a goat's skin, or to wear it, and to put one foot upon another, or one hand upon another; for all these things are held to be hindrances to the cure. All these they enjoin with reference to its divinity, as if possessed of more knowledge, and announcing beforehand other causes so that if the person should recover, theirs would be the honor and credit; and if he should die, they would have a certain defense, as if the gods, and not they, were to blame, seeing they had administered nothing either to eat or drink as medicines, nor had overheated him with baths, so as to prove the cause of what had happened. But I am of opinion that (if this were true) none of the Libyans, who live in the interior, would be free from this disease, since they all sleep on goats' skins, and live upon goats' flesh; neither have they couch, robe, nor shoe that is not made of goat's skin, for they have no other herds but goats and oxen. But if these things, when administered in food, aggravate the disease, and if it be cured by abstinence from them, godhead is not the cause at all; nor will purifications be of any avail, but it is the food which is beneficial and prejudicial, and the influence of the divinity vanishes.

Thus, they who try to cure these maladies in this way, appear to me neither to reckon them sacred nor divine. For when they are removed by such purifications, and this method of cure, what is to prevent them from being brought upon men and induced by other devices similar to these? So that the cause is no longer divine, but human. For whoever is able, by purifications conjurations, to drive away such an affection, will be able, by other practices, to excite it; and, according to this view, its divine nature is entirely done away with. By such sayings and doings, they profess to be possessed of superior knowledge, and deceive mankind by enjoining lustrations and purifications upon them, while their discourse turns upon the divinity and the godhead. And yet it would appear to me that their discourse savors not of piety, as they suppose, but rather of impiety, and as if there were no gods, and that what they hold to be holy and divine, were impious and unholy. This I will now explain.

For, if they profess to know how to bring down the moon, darken the sun, induce storms and fine weather, and rains and droughts, and make the sea and land unproductive, and so forth, whether they arrogate this power as being derived from mysteries or any other knowledge or consideration, they appear to me to practice impiety, and either to fancy that there are no gods, or, if there are, that they have no ability to ward off any of the greatest evils. How, then, are they not enemies to the gods? For if a man by magical arts and sacrifices will bring down the moon, and darken the sun, and induce storms, or fine weather, I should not believe that there was anything divine, but human, in these things, provided the power of the divine were overpowered by human knowledge and subjected to it. But perhaps it will be said, these things are not so, but, not withstanding, men being in want of the means of life, invent many and various things, and devise many contrivances for all other things, and for this disease, in every phase of the disease, assigning the cause to a god. Nor do they remember the same things once, but frequently. For, if they imitate a goat, or grind their teeth, or if their right side be convulsed, they say that the mother of the gods is the cause. But if they speak in a sharper and more intense tone, they resemble this state to a horse, and say that Poseidon is the cause. Or if any excrement be passed, which is often the case, owing to the violence of the disease, the appellation of Enodia is adhibited; or, if it be passed in smaller and denser masses, like bird's, it is said to be from Apollo Nomius. But if foam be emitted by the mouth, and the patient kick with his feet, Ares then gets the blame. But terrors which happen during the night, and fevers, and delirium, and jumpings out of bed, and frightful apparitions, and fleeing away,—all these they hold to be the plots of Hecate, and the invasions the and use purifications and incantations, and, as appears to me, make the divinity to be most wicked and most impious. For they purify those laboring under this disease, with the same sorts of blood and the other means that are used in the case of those who are stained with crimes, and of malefactors, or who have been enchanted by men, or who have done any wicked act; who ought to do the very reverse, namely, sacrifice and pray, and, bringing gifts to the temples, supplicate the gods. But now they do none of these things, but purify; and some of the purifications they conceal in the earth, and some they throw into the sea, and some they carry to the mountains where no one can touch or tread upon them. But these they ought to take to the temples and present to the god, if a god be the cause of the disease. Neither truly do I count it a worthy opinion to hold that the body of man is polluted by god, the most impure by the most holy; for were it defiled, or did it suffer from any other thing, it would be like to be purified and sanctified rather than polluted by god. For it is the divinity which purifies and sanctifies the greatest of offenses and the most wicked, and which proves our protection from them. And we mark out the boundaries of the temples and the groves of the gods, so that no one may pass them unless he be pure, and when we enter them we are sprinkled with holy water, not as being polluted, but as laying aside any other pollution which we formerly had. And thus it appears to me to hold, with regard to purifications.

But this disease seems to me to be no more divine than others; but it has its nature such as other diseases have, and a cause whence it originates, and its nature and cause are divine only just as much as all others are, and it is curable no less than the others, unless when, the from of time, it is confirmed, and has became stronger than the remedies applied. Its origin is hereditary, like that of other diseases. For if a phlegmatic person be born of a phlegmatic, and a bilious of a bilious, and a phthisical of a phthisical, and one having spleen disease, of another having disease of the spleen, what is to hinder it from happening that where the father and mother were subject to this disease, certain of their offspring should be so affected also? As the semen comes from all parts of the body, healthy particles will come from healthy parts, and unhealthy from unhealthy parts. And another great proof that it is in nothing more divine than other diseases is, that it occurs in those who are of a phlegmatic constitution, but does not attack the bilious. Yet, if it were more divine than the others, this disease ought to befall all alike, and make no distinction between the bilious and phlegmatic.

But the brain is the cause of this affection, as it is of other very great diseases, and in what manner and from what cause it is formed, I will now plainly declare. The brain of man, as in all other animals, is double, and a thin membrane divides it through the middle, and therefore the pain is not always in the same part of the head; for sometimes it is situated on either side, and sometimes the whole is affected; and veins run toward it from all parts of the body, many of which are small, but two are thick, the one from the liver, and the other from the spleen. And it is thus with regard to the one from the liver: a portion of it runs downward through the parts on the side, near the kidneys and the psoas muscles, to the inner part of the thigh, and extends to the foot. It is called vena cava. The other runs upward by the right veins and the lungs, and divides into branches for the heart and the right arm. The remaining part of it rises upward across the clavicle to the right side of the neck, and is superficial so as to be seen; near the ear it is concealed, and there it divides; its thickest, largest, and most hollow part ends in the brain; another small vein goes to the right ear, another to the right eye, and another to the nostril. Such are the distributions of the hepatic vein. And a vein from the spleen is distributed on the left side, upward and downward, like that from the liver, but more slender and feeble.

By these veins we draw in much breath, since they are the spiracles of our bodies inhaling air to themselves and distributing it to the rest of the body, and to the smaller veins, and they and afterwards exhale it. For the breath cannot be stationary, but it passes upward and downward, for if stopped and intercepted, the part where it is stopped becomes powerless. In proof of this, when, in sitting or lying, the small veins are compressed, so that the breath from the larger vein does not pass into them, the part is immediately seized with numbness; and it is so likewise with regard to the other veins.

This malady, then, affects phlegmatic people, but not bilious. It begins to be formed while the foetus is still in utero. For the brain, like the other organs, is depurated and grows before birth. If, then, in this purgation it be properly and moderately depurated, and neither more nor less than what is proper be secreted from it, the head is thus in the most healthy condition. If the secretion (melting) the from the brain be greater than natural, the person, when he grows up, will have his head diseased, and full of noises, and will neither be able to endure the sun nor cold. Or, if the melting take place from any one part, either from the eye or ear, or if a vein has become slender, that part will be deranged in proportion to the melting. Or, should depuration not take place, but congestion accumulate in the brain, it necessarily becomes phlegmatic. And such children as have an eruption of ulcers on the head, on the ears, and along the rest of the body, with copious discharges of saliva and mucus,—these, in after life, enjoy best health; for in this way the phlegm which ought to have been purged off in the womb, is discharged and cleared away, and persons so purged, for the most part, are not subject to attacks of this disease. But such as have had their skin free from eruptions, and have had no discharge of saliva or mucus, nor have undergone the proper purgation in the womb, these persons run the risk of being seized with this disease.

But should the defluxion make its way to the heart, the person is seized with palpitation and asthma, the chest becomes diseased, and some also have curvature of the spine. For when a defluxion of cold phlegm takes place on the lungs and heart, the blood is chilled, and the veins, being violently chilled, palpitate in the lungs and heart, and the heart palpitates, so that from this necessity asthma and orthopnoea supervene. For it does not receive the spirits as much breath as he needs until the defluxion of phlegm be mastered, and being heated is distributed to the veins, then it ceases from its palpitation and difficulty of breathing, and this takes place as soon as it obtains an abundant supply; and this will be more slowly, provided the defluxion be more abundant, or if it be less, more quickly. And if the defluxions be more condensed, the epileptic attacks will be more frequent, but otherwise if it be rarer. Such are the symptoms when the defluxion is upon the lungs and heart; but if it be upon the bowels, the person is attacked with diarrhoea.

And if, being shut out from all these outlets, its defluxion be determined to the veins I have formerly mentioned, the patient loses his speech, and chokes, and foam issues by the mouth, the teeth are fixed, the hands are contracted, the eyes distorted, he becomes insensible, and in some cases the bowels are evacuated. And these symptoms occur sometimes on the left side, sometimes on the right, and sometimes in both. The cause of everyone of these symptoms I will now explain. The man becomes speechless when the phlegm, suddenly descending into the veins, shuts out the air, and does not admit it either to the brain or to the vena cava, or to the ventricles, but interrupts the inspiration. For when a person draws in air by the mouth and nostrils, the breath goes first to the brain, then the greater part of it to the internal cavity, and part to the lungs, and part to the veins, and from them it is distributed to the other parts of the body along the veins; and whatever passes to the stomach cools, and does nothing more; and so also with regard to the lungs. But the air which enters the veins is of use (to the body) by entering the brain and its ventricles, and thus it imparts sensibility and motion to all the members, so that when the veins are excluded from the air by the phlegm and do not receive it, the man loses his speech and intellect, and the hands become powerless, and are contracted, the blood stopping and not being diffused, as it was wont; and the eyes are distorted owing to the veins being excluded from the air; and they palpitate; and froth from the lungs issues by the mouth. For when the breath does not find entrance to him, he foams and sputters like a dying person. And the bowels are evacuated in consequence of the violent suffocation; and the suffocation is produced when the liver and stomach ascend to the diaphragm, and the mouth of the stomach is shut up; this takes place when the breath does not enter by the mouth, as it is wont. The patient kicks with his feet when the air is shut up in the lungs and cannot find an outlet, owing to the phlegm; and rushing by the blood upward and downward, it occasions convulsions and pain, and therefore he kicks with his feet. All these symptoms he endures when the cold phlegm passes into the warm blood, for it congeals and stops the blood. And if the deflexion be copious and thick, it immediately proves fatal to him, for by its cold it prevails over the blood and congeals it; or, if it be less, it in the first place obtains the mastery, and stops the respiration; and then in the course of time, when it is diffused along the veins and mixed with much warm blood, it is thus overpowered, the veins receive the air, and the patient recovers his senses.

Of little children who are seized with this disease, the greater part die, provided the defluxion be copious and humid, for the veins being slender cannot admit the phlegm, owing to its thickness and abundance; but the blood is cooled and congealed, and the child immediately dies. But if the phlegm be in small quantity, and make a defluxion into both the veins, or to those on either side, the children survive, but exhibit notable marks of the disorder; for either the mouth is drawn aside, or an eye, the neck, or a hand, wherever a vein being filled with phlegm loses its tone, and is attenuated, and the part of the body connected with this vein is necessarily rendered weaker and defective. But for the most it affords relief for a longer interval; for the child is no longer seized with these attacks, if once it has contracted this impress of the disease, in consequence of which the other veins are necessarily affected, and to a certain degree attenuated, so as just to admit the air, but no longer to permit the influx of phlegm. However, the parts are proportionally enfeebled whenever the veins are in an unhealthy state. When in striplings the defluxion is small and to the right side, they recover without leaving any marks of the disease, but there is danger of its becoming habitual, and even increasing if not treated by suitable remedies. Thus, or very nearly so, is the case when it attacks children.

To persons of a more advanced age, it neither proves fatal, nor produces distortions. For their veins are capacious and are filled with hot blood; and therefore the phlegm can neither prevail nor cool the blood, so as to coagulate it, but it is quickly overpowered and mixed with the blood, and thus the veins receive the air, and sensibility remains; and, owing to their strength, the aforesaid symptoms are less likely to seize them. But when this disease attacks very old people, it therefore proves fatal, or induces paraplegia, because the veins are empty, and the blood scanty, thin, and watery. When, therefore, the defluxion is copious, and the season winter, it proves fatal; for it chokes up the exhalents, and coagulates the blood if the defluxion be to both sides; but if to either, it merely induces paraplegia. For the blood being thin, cold, and scanty, cannot prevail over the but being itself overpowered, it is coagulated, so that those parts in which the blood is corrupted, lose their strength.

The flux is to the right rather than to the left because the veins there are more capacious and numerous than on the left side, for on the one side they spring from the liver, and on the other from the spleen. The defluxion and melting down take place most especially in the case of children in whom the head is heated either by the sun or by fire, or if the brain suddenly contract a rigor, and then the phlegm is excreted. For it is melted down by the heat and diffusion of the but it is excreted by the congealing and contracting of it, and thus a defluxion takes place. And in some this is the cause of the disease, and in others, when the south wind quickly succeeds to northern breezes, it suddenly unbinds and relaxes the brain, which is contracted and weak, so that there is an inundation of phlegm, and thus the defluxion takes place. The defluxion also takes place in consequence of fear, from any hidden cause, if we are the at any person's calling aloud, or while crying, when one cannot quickly recover one's breath, such as often happens to children. When any of these things occur, the body immediately shivers, the person becoming speechless cannot draw his breath, but the breath (pneuma) stops, the brain is contracted, the blood stands still, and thus the excretion and defluxion of the phlegm take place. In children, these are the causes of the attack at first. But to old persons winter is most inimical. For when the head and brain have been heated at a great fire, and then the person is brought into cold and has a rigor, or when from cold he comes into warmth, and sits at the fire, he is apt to suffer in the same way, and thus he is seized in the manner described above. And there is much danger of the same thing occurring, if his head be exposed to the sun, but less so in summer, as the changes are not sudden. When a person has passed the twentieth year of his life, this disease is not apt to seize him, unless it has become habitual from childhood, or at least this is rarely or never the case. For the veins are filled with blood, and the brain consistent and firm, so that it does not run down into the veins, or if it do, it does not master the blood, which is copious and hot.

But when it has gained strength from one's childhood, and become habitual, such a person usually suffers attacks, and is seized with them in changes of the winds, especially in south winds, and it is difficult of removal. For the brain becomes more humid than natural, and is inundated with phlegm, so that the defluxions become more frequent, and the phlegm can no longer be the nor the brain be dried up, but it becomes wet and humid. This you may ascertain in particular, from beasts of the flock which are seized with this disease, and more especially goats, for they are most frequently attacked with it. If you will cut open the head, you will find the brain humid, full of sweat, and having a bad smell. And in this way truly you may see that it is not a god that injures the body, but disease. And so it is with man. For when the disease has prevailed for a length of time, it is no longer curable, as the brain is corroded by the phlegm, and melted, and what is melted down becomes water, and surrounds the brain externally, and overflows it; wherefore they are more frequently and readily seized with the disease. And therefore the disease is protracted, because the influx is thin, owing to its quantity, and is immediately overpowered by the blood and heated all through.

But such persons as are habituated to the disease know beforehand when they are about to be seized and flee from men; if their own house be at hand, they run home, but if not, to a deserted place, where as few persons as possible will see them falling, and they immediately cover themselves up. This they do from shame of the affection, and not from fear of the divinity, as many suppose. And little children at first fall down wherever they may happen to be, from inexperience. But when they have been often seized, and feel its approach beforehand, they flee to their mothers, or to any other person they are acquainted with, from terror and dread of the affection, for being still infants they do not know yet what it is to be ashamed.

Therefore, they are attacked during changes of the winds, and especially south winds, then also with north winds, and afterwards also with the others. These are the strongest winds, and the most opposed to one another, both as to direction and power. For, the north wind condenses the air, and separates from it whatever is muddy and nebulous, and renders it clearer and brighter, and so in like manner also, all the winds which arise from the sea and other waters; for they extract the humidity and nebulosity from all objects, and from men themselves, and therefore it (the north wind) is the most wholesome of the winds. But the effects of the south are the very reverse. For in the first place it begins by melting and diffusing the condensed air, and therefore it does not blow strong at first, but is gentle at the commencement, because it is not able at once to overcome the and compacted air, which yet in a while it dissolves. It produces the same effects upon the land, the sea, the fountains, the wells, and on every production which contains humidity, and this, there is in all things, some more, some less. For all these feel the effects of this wind, and from clear they become cloudy, from cold, hot; from dry, moist; and whatever ear then vessels are placed upon the ground, filled with wine or any other fluid, are affected with the south wind, and undergo a change. And the a change. And the sun, and the moon, it renders blunter appearance than they naturally are. When, then, it possesses such powers over things so great and strong, and the body is made to feel and undergo changes in the changes of the winds, it necessarily follows that the brain should be disolved and overpowered with moisture, and that the veins should become more relaxed by the south winds, and that by the north the healthiest portion of the brain should become contracted, while the most morbid and humid is secreted, and overflows externally, and that catarrhs should thus take place in the changes of these winds. Thus is this disease formed and prevails from those things which enter into and go out of the body, and it is not more difficult to understand or to cure than the others, neither is it more divine than other diseases.

Men ought to know that from nothing else but the brain come joys, delights, laughter and sports, and sorrows, griefs, despondency, and lamentations. And by this, in an especial manner, we acquire wisdom and knowledge, and see and hear, and know what are foul and what are fair, what are bad and what are good, what are sweet, and what unsavory; some we discriminate by habit, and some we perceive by their utility. By this we distinguish objects of relish and disrelish, according to the seasons; and the same things do not always please us. And by the same organ we become mad and delirious, and fears and terrors assail us, some by night, and some by day, and dreams and untimely wanderings, and cares that are not suitable, and ignorance of present circumstances, desuetude, and unskilfulness. All these things we endure from the brain, when it is not healthy, but is more hot, more cold, more moist, or more dry than natural, or when it suffers any other preternatural and unusual affection. And we become mad from its humidity. For when it is more moist than natural, it is necessarily put into motion, and the affection being moved, neither the sight nor hearing can be at rest, and the tongue speaks in accordance with the sight and hearing.

As long as the brain is at rest, the man enjoys his reason, but the depravement of the brain arises from phlegm and bile, either of which you may recognize in this manner: Those who are mad from phlegm are quiet, and do not cry out nor make a noise; but those from bile are vociferous, malignant, and will not be quiet, but are always doing something improper. If the madness be constant, these are the causes thereof. But if terrors and fears assail, they are connected with derangement of the brain, and derangement is owing to its being heated. And it is heated by bile when it is determined to the brain along the bloodvessels running from the trunk; and fear is present until it returns again to the veins and trunk, when it ceases. He is grieved and troubled when the brain is unseasonably cooled and contracted beyond its wont. This it suffers from phlegm, and from the same affection the patient becomes oblivious. He calls out and screams at night when the brain is suddenly heated. The bilious endure this. But the phlegmatic are not heated, except when much blood goes to the brain, and creates an ebullition. Much blood passes along the aforesaid veins. But when the man happens to see a frightful dream and is in fear as if awake, then his face is in a greater glow, and the eyes are red when the patient is in fear. And the understanding meditates doing some mischief, and thus it is affected in sleep. But if, when awakened, he returns to himself, and the blood is again distributed along the veins, it ceases.

In these ways I am of the opinion that the brain exercises the greatest power in the man. This is the interpreter to us of those things which emanate from the air, when the brain happens to be in a sound state. But the air supplies sense to it. And the eyes, the ears, the tongue and the feet, administer such things as the brain cogitates. For in as much as it is supplied with air, does it impart sense to the body. It is the brain which is the messenger to the understanding. For when the man draws the breath into himself, it passes first to the brain, and thus the air is distributed to the rest of the body, leaving in the brain its acme, and whatever has sense and understanding. For if it passed first to the body and last to the brain, then having left in the flesh and veins the judgment, when it reached the brain it would be hot, and not at all pure, but mixed with the humidity from flesh and blood, so as to be no longer pure.

Wherefore, I say, that it is the brain which interprets the understanding. But the diaphragm has obtained its name (frenes) from accident and usage, and not from reality or nature, for I know no power which it possesses, either as to sense or understanding, except that when the man is affected with unexpected joy or sorrow, it throbs and produces palpitations, owing to its thinness, and as having no belly to receive anything good or bad that may present themselves to it, but it is thrown into commotion by both these, from its natural weakness. It then perceives beforehand none of those things which occur in the body, but has received its name vaguely and without any proper reason, like the parts about the heart, which are called auricles, but which contribute nothing towards hearing. Some say that we think with the heart, and that this is the part which is grieved, and experiences care. But it is not so; only it contracts like the diaphragm, and still more so for the same causes. For veins from all parts of the body run to it, and it has valves, so as to as to perceive if any pain or pleasurable emotion befall the man. For when grieved the body necessarily shudders, and is contracted, and from excessive joy it is affected in like manner. Wherefore the heart and the diaphragm are particularly sensitive, they have nothing to do, however, with the operations of the understanding, but of all but of all these the brain is the cause. Since, then, the brain, as being the primary seat of sense and of the spirits, perceives whatever occurs in the body, if any change more powerful than usual take place in the air, owing to the seasons, the brain becomes changed by the state of the air. For, on this account, the brain first perceives, because, I say, all the most acute, most powerful, and most deadly diseases, and those which are most difficult to be understood by the inexperienced, fall upon the brain.

And the disease called the Sacred arises from causes as the others, namely, those things which enter and quit the body, such as cold, the sun, and the winds, which are ever changing and are never at rest. And these things are divine, so that there is no necessity for making a distinction, and holding this disease to be more divine than the others, but all are divine, and all human. And each has its own peculiar nature and power, and none is of an ambiguous nature, or irremediable. And the most of them are curable by the same means as those by which any other thing is food to one, and injurious to another. Thus, then, the physician should understand and distinguish the season of each, so that at one time he may attend to the nourishment and increase, and at another to abstraction and diminution. And in this disease as in all others, he must strive not to feed the disease, but endeavor to wear it out by administering whatever is most opposed to each disease, and not that which favors and is allied to it. For by that which is allied to it, it gains vigor and increase, but it wears out and disappears under the use of that which is opposed to it. But whoever is acquainted with such a change in men, and can render a man humid and dry, hot and cold by regimen, could also cure this disease, if he recognizes the proper season for administering his remedies, without minding purifications, spells, and all other illiberal practices of a like kind.

ON AIRS, WATERS, AND PLACES

WHOEVER wishes to investigate medicine properly, should proceed thus: in the first place to consider the seasons of the year, and what effects each of them produces for they are not at all alike, but differ much from themselves in regard to their changes. Then the winds, the hot and the cold, especially such as are common to all countries, and then such as are peculiar to each locality. We must also consider the qualities of the waters, for as they differ from one another in taste and weight, so also do they differ much in their qualities. In the same manner, when one comes into a city to which he is a stranger, he ought to consider its situation, how it lies as to the winds and the rising of the sun; for its influence is not the same whether it lies to the north or the south, to the rising or to the setting sun. These things one ought to consider most attentively, and concerning the waters which the inhabitants use, whether they be marshy and soft, or hard, and running from elevated and rocky situations, and then if saltish and unfit for cooking; and the ground, whether it be naked and deficient in water, or wooded and well watered, and whether it lies in a hollow, confined situation, or is elevated and cold; and the mode in which the inhabitants live, and what are their pursuits, whether they are fond of drinking and eating to excess, and given to indolence, or are fond of exercise and labor, and not given to excess in eating and drinking.

2. From these things he must proceed to investigate everything else. For if one knows all these things well, or at least the greater part of them, he cannot miss knowing, when he comes into a strange city, either the diseases peculiar to the place, or the particular nature of common diseases, so that he will not be in doubt as to the treatment of the diseases, or commit mistakes, as is likely to be the case provided one had not previously considered these matters. And in particular, as the season and the year advances, he can tell what epidemic diseases will attack the city, either in summer or in winter, and what each individual will be in danger of experiencing from the change of regimen. For knowing the changes of the seasons, the risings and settings of the stars, how each of them takes place, he will be able to know beforehand what sort of a year is going to ensue. Having made these investigations, and knowing beforehand the seasons, such a one must be acquainted with each particular, and must succeed in the preservation of health, and be by no means unsuccessful in the practice of his art. And if it shall be thought that these things belong rather to meteorology, it will be admitted, on second thoughts, that astronomy contributes not a little, but a very great deal, indeed, to medicine. For with the seasons the digestive organs of men undergo a change.

3. But how of the aforementioned things should be investigated and explained, I will now declare in a clear manner. A city that is exposed to hot winds (these are between the wintry rising, and the wintry setting of the sun), and to which these are peculiar, but which is sheltered from the north winds; in such a city the waters will be plenteous and saltish, and as they run from an elevated source, they are necessarily hot in summer, and cold in winter; the heads of the inhabitants are of a humid and pituitous constitution, and their bellies subject to frequent disorders, owing to the phlegm running down from the head; the forms of their bodies, for the most part, are rather flabby; they do not eat nor drink much; drinking wine in particular, and more especially if carried to intoxication, is oppressive to them; and the following diseases are peculiar to the district: in the first place, the women are sickly and subject to excessive menstruation; then many are unfruitful from disease, and not from nature, and they have frequent miscarriages; infants are subject to attacks of convulsions and asthma, which they consider to be connected with infancy, and hold to be a sacred disease (epilepsy). The men are subject to attacks of dysentery, diarrhea, hepialus, chronic fevers in winter, of epinyctis, frequently, and of hemorrhoids about the anus. Pleurisies, peripneumonies, ardent fevers, and whatever diseases are reckoned acute, do not often occur, for such diseases are not apt to prevail where the bowels are loose. Ophthalmies occur of a humid character, but not of a serious nature, and of short duration, unless they attack epidemically from the change of the seasons. And when they pass their fiftieth year, defluxions supervening from the brain, render them paralytic when exposed suddenly to strokes of the sun, or to cold. These diseases are endemic to them, and, moreover, if any epidemic disease connected with the change of the seasons, prevail, they are also liable to it.

4. But the following is the condition of cities which have the opposite exposure, namely, to cold winds, between the summer settings and the summer risings of the sun, and to which these winds are peculiar, and which are sheltered from the south and the hot breezes. In the first place the waters are, for the most part, hard cold. The men must necessarily be well braced and slender, and they must have the discharges downwards of the alimentary canal hard, and of difficult evacuation, while those upwards are more fluid, and rather bilious than pituitous. Their heads are sound and hard, and they are liable to burstings (of vessels?) for the most part. The diseases which prevail epidemically with them, are pleurisies, and those which are called acute diseases. This must be the case when the bowels are bound; and from any causes, many become affected with suppurations in the lungs, the cause of which is the tension of the body, and hardness of the bowels; for their dryness and the coldness of the water dispose them to ruptures (of vessels?). Such constitutions must be given to excess of eating, but not of drinking; for it is not possible to be gourmands and drunkards at the same time. Ophthalmies, too, at length supervene; these being of a hard and violent nature, and soon ending in rupture of the eyes; persons under thirty years of age are liable to severe bleedings at the nose in summer; attacks of epilepsy are rare but severe. Such people are likely to be rather long-lived; their ulcers are not attended with serious discharges, nor of a malignant character; in disposition they are rather ferocious than gentle. The diseases I have mentioned are peculiar to the men, and besides they are liable to any common complaint which may be prevailing from the changes of the seasons. But the women, in the first place, are of a hard constitution, from the waters being hard, indigestible, and cold; and their menstrual discharges are not regular, but in small quantity, and painful. Then they have difficult parturition, but are not very subject to abortions. And when they do bring forth children, they are unable to nurse them; for the hardness and indigestable nature of the water puts away their milk. Phthisis frequently supervenes after childbirth, for the efforts of it frequently bring on ruptures and strains. Children while still little are subject to dropsies in the testicle, which disappear as they grow older; in such a town they are late in attaining manhood. It is, as I have now stated, with regard to hot and cold winds and cities thus exposed.

5. Cities that are exposed to winds between the summer and the winter risings of the sun, and those the opposite to them, have the following characters:—Those which lie to the rising of the sun are all likely to be more healthy than such as are turned to the North, or those exposed to the hot winds, even if there should not be a furlong between them. In the first place, both the heat and cold are more moderate. Then such waters as flow to the rising sun, must necessarily be clear, fragrant, soft, and delightful to drink, in such a city. For the sun in rising and shining upon them purifies them, by dispelling the vapors which generally prevail in the morning. The persons of the inhabitants are, for the most part, well colored and blooming, unless some disease counteract. The inhabitants have clear voices, and in temper and intellect are superior to those which are exposed to the north, and all the productions of the country in like manner are better. A city so situated resembles the spring as to moderation between heat and cold, and the diseases are few in number, and of a feeble kind, and bear a resemblance to the diseases which prevail in regions exposed to hot winds. The women there are very prolific, and have easy deliveries. Thus it is with regard to them.

6. But such cities as lie to the west, and which are sheltered from winds blowing from the east, and which the hot winds and the cold winds of the north scarcely touch, must necessarily be in a very unhealthy situation: in the first place the waters are not clear, the cause of which is, because the mist prevails commonly in the morning, and it is mixed up with the water and destroys its clearness, for the sun does not shine upon the water until he be considerably raised above the horizon. And in summer, cold breezes from the east blow and dews fall; and in the latter part

of the day the setting sun particularly scorches the inhabitants, and therefore they are pale and enfeebled, and are partly subject to all the aforesaid diseases, but no one is peculiar to them. Their voices are rough and hoarse owing to the state of the air, which in such a situation is generally impure and unwholesome, for they have not the northern winds to purify it; and these winds they have are of a very humid character, such being the nature of the evening breezes. Such a situation of a city bears a great resemblance to autumn as regards the changes of the day, inasmuch as the difference between morning and evening is great. So it is with regard to the winds that are conducive to health, or the contrary.

7. And I wish to give an account of the other kinds of waters, namely, of such as are wholesome and such as are unwholesome, and what bad and what good effects may be derived from water; for water contributes much towards health. Such waters then as are marshy, stagnant, and belong to lakes, are necessarily hot in summer, thick, and have a strong smell, since they have no current; but being constantly supplied by rain-water, and the sun heating them, they necessarily want their proper color, are unwholesome and form bile; in winter, they become congealed, cold, and muddy with the snow and ice, so that they are most apt to engender phlegm, and bring on hoarseness; those who drink them have large and obstructed spleens, their bellies are hard, emaciated, and hot; and their shoulders, collar-bones, and faces are emaciated; for their flesh is melted down and taken up by the spleen, and hence they are slender; such persons then are voracious and thirsty; their bellies are very dry both above and below, so that they require the strongest medicines. This disease is habitual to them both in summer and in winter, and in addition they are very subject to dropsies of a most fatal character;

and in summer dysenteries, diarrheas, and protracted quartan fevers frequently seize them, and these diseases when prolonged dispose such constitutions to dropsies, and thus prove fatal. These are the diseases which attack them in summer; but in winter younger persons are liable to pneumonia, and maniacal affections; and older persons to ardent fevers, from hardness of the belly. Women are subject to oedema and leucophlegmasiae; when pregnant they have difficult deliveries; their infants are large and swelled, and then during nursing they become wasted and sickly, and the lochial discharge after parturition does not proceed properly with the women. The children are particularly subject to hernia, and adults to varices and ulcers on their legs, so that persons with such constitutions cannot be long-lived, but before the usual period they fall into a state of premature old age. And further, the women appear to be with child, and when the time of parturition arrives, the fulness of the belly disappears, and this happens from dropsy of the uterus. Such waters then I reckon bad for every purpose. The next to them in badness are those which have their fountains in rocks, so that they must necessarily be hard, or come from a soil which produces thermal waters, such as those having iron, copper, silver, gold, sulphur, alum, bitumen, or nitre (soda) in them; for all these are formed by the force of heat. Good waters cannot proceed from such a soil, but those that are hard and of a heating nature, difficult to pass by urine, and of difficult evacuation by the bowels. The best are those which flow from elevated grounds, and hills of earth; these are sweet, clear, and can bear a little wine; they are hot in summer and cold in winter, for such necessarily must be the waters from deep wells. But those are most to be commended which run to the rising of the sun, and especially to the summer sun; for such are necessarily more clear, fragrant, and light. But all such as are salty, crude, and harsh, are not good for drink. But there are certain constitutions and diseases with which such waters agree when drunk, as I will explain presently. Their characters are as follows: the best are such as have their fountains to the east; the next, those between the summer risings and settings of the sun, and especially those to the risings; and third, those between the summer and winter settings; but the worst are those to the south, and the parts between the winter rising and setting, and those to the south are very bad, but those to the north are better. They are to be used as follows: whoever is in good health and strength need not mind, but may always drink whatever is at hand. But whoever wishes to drink the most suitable for any disease, may accomplish his purpose by attending to the following directions: To persons whose bellies are hard and easily burnt up, the sweetest, the lightest, and the most limpid waters will be proper; but those persons whose bellies are soft, loose, and pituitous, should choose the hardest, those kinds that are most crude, and the saltiest, for thus will they be most readily dried up; for such waters as are adapted for boiling, and are of a very solvent nature, naturally loosen readily and melt down the bowels; but such as are intractable, hard, and by no means proper for boiling, these rather bind and dry up the bowels. People have deceived themselves with regard to salt waters, from inexperience, for they think these waters purgative, whereas they are the very reverse; for such waters are crude, and ill adapted for boiling, so that the belly is more likely to be bound up than loosened by them. And thus it is with regard to the waters of springs.

8. I will now tell how it is with respect to rain-water, and water from snow. Rain waters, then, are the lightest, the sweetest, the thinnest, and the clearest; for originally the sun raises and attracts the thinnest and lightest part of the water, as is obvious from the nature of salts; for the saltish part is left behind owing to its thickness and weight, and forms salts; but the sun attracts the thinnest part, owing to its lightness, and he abstracts this not only from the lakes, but also from the sea, and from all things which contain humidity, and there is humidity in everything; and from man himself the sun draws off the thinnest and lightest part of the juices. As a strong proof of this, when a man walks in the sun, or sits down having a garment on, whatever parts of the body the sun shines upon do not sweat, for the sun carries off whatever sweat makes its appearance; but those parts which are covered by the garment, or anything else, sweat, for the particles of sweat are drawn and forced out by the sun, and are preserved by the cover so as not to be dissipated by the sun; but when the person comes into the shade the whole body equally perspires, because the sun no longer shines upon it. Wherefore, of all kinds of water, these spoil the soonest; and rain water has a bad spot smell, because its particles are collected and mixed together from most objects, so as to spoil the soonest. And in addition to this, when attracted and raised up, being carried about and mixed with the air, whatever part of it is turbid and darkish is separated and removed from the other, and becomes cloud and mist, but the most attenuated and lightest part is left, and becomes sweet, being heated and concocted by the sun, for all other things when concocted become sweet. While dissipated then and not in a state of consistence it is carried aloft. But when collected and condensed by contrary winds, it falls down wherever it happens to be most condensed. For this is likely to happen when the clouds being carried along and moving with a wind which does not allow them to rest, suddenly encounters another wind and other clouds from the opposite direction: there it is first condensed, and what is behind is carried up to the spot, and thus it thickens, blackens, and is conglomerated, and by its weight it falls down and becomes rain. Such, to all appearance, are the best of waters, but they require to be boiled and strained; for otherwise they have a bad smell, and occasion hoarseness and thickness of the voice to those who drink them. Those from snow and ice are all bad, for when once congealed, they never again recover their former nature; for whatever is clear, light, and sweet in them, is separated and disappears; but the most turbid and weightiest part is left behind. You may ascertain this in the following manner: If in winter you will pour water by measure into a vessel and expose it to the open air until it is all frozen, and then on the following day bring it into a warm situation where the ice will thaw, if you will measure the water again when dissolved you will find it much less in quantity. This is a proof that the lightest and thinnest part is dissipated and dried up by the congelation, and not the heaviest and thickest, for that is impossible: wherefore I hold that waters from snow and ice, and those allied to them, are the worst of any for all purposes whatever. Such are the characters of rain-water, and those from ice and snow.

9. Men become affected with the stone, and are seized with diseases of the kidneys, strangury, sciatica, and become ruptured, when they drink all sorts of waters, and those from great rivers into which other rivulets run, or from a lake into which many streams of all sorts flow, and such as are brought from a considerable distance. For it is impossible that such waters can resemble one another, but one kind is sweet, another saltish and aluminous, and some flow from thermal springs; and these being all mixed up together disagree, and the strongest part always prevails; but the same kind is not always the strongest, but sometimes one and sometimes another, according to the winds, for the north wind imparts strength to this water, and the south to that, and so also with regard to the others. There must be deposits of mud and sand in the vessels from such waters, and the aforesaid diseases must be engendered by them when drunk, but why not to all I will now explain. When the bowels are loose and in a healthy state, and when the bladder is not hot, nor the neck of the bladder very contracted, all such persons pass water freely, and no concretion forms in the bladder; but those in whom the belly is hot, the bladder must be in the same condition; and when preternaturally heated, its neck becomes inflamed; and when these things happen, the bladder does not expel the urine, but raises its heat excessively. And the thinnest part of it is secreted, and the purest part is passed off in the form of urine, but the thickest and most turbid part is condensed and concreted, at first in small quantity, but afterwards in greater; for being rolled about in the urine, whatever is of a thick consistence it assimilates to itself, and thus it increases and becomes indurated. And when such persons make water, the stone forced down by the urine falls into the neck of the bladder and stops the urine, and occasions intense pain; so that calculous children rub their privy parts and tear at them, as supposing that the obstruction to the urine is situated there. As a proof that it is as I say, persons affected with calculus have very limpid urine, because the thickest and foulest part remains and is concreted. Thus it generally is in cases of calculus. It forms also in children from milk, when it is not wholesome, but very hot and bilious, for it heats the bowels and bladder, so that the urine being also heated undergoes the same change. And I hold that it is better to give children only the most diluted wine, for such will least burn up and dry the veins. Calculi do not form so readily in women, for in them the urethra is short and wide, so that in them the urine is easily expelled; neither do they rub the pudendum with their hands, nor handle the passage like males; for the urethra in women opens direct into the pudendum, which is not the case with men, neither in them is the urethra so wide, and they drink more than children do. Thus, or nearly so, is it with regard to them.

10. And respecting the seasons, one may judge whether the year will prove sickly or healthy from the following observations: —If the appearances connected with the rising and setting stars be as they should be; if there be rains in autumn; if the winter be mild, neither very tepid nor unseasonably cold, and if in spring the rains be seasonable, and so also in summer, the year is likely to prove healthy. But if the winter be dry and northerly, and the spring showery and southerly, the summer will necessarily be of a febrile character, and give rise to ophthalmies and dysenteries. For when suffocating heat sets in all of a sudden, while the earth is moistened by the vernal showers, and by the south wind, the heat is necessarily doubled from the earth, which is thus soaked by rain and heated by a burning sun, while, at the same time, men's bellies are not in an orderly state, nor the brain properly dried; for it is impossible, after such a spring, but that the body and its flesh must be loaded with humors, so that very acute fevers will attack all, but especially those of a phlegmatic constitution. Dysenteries are also likely to occur to women and those of a very humid temperament. And if at the rising of the Dogstar rain and wintery storms supervene, and if the etesian winds blow, there is reason to hope that these diseases will cease, and that the autumn will be healthy; but if not, it is likely to be a fatal season to children and women, but least of all to old men; and that convalescents will pass into quartans, and from quartans into dropsies; but if the winter be southerly, showery and mild, but the spring northerly, dry, and of a wintry character, in the first place women who happen to be with child, and whose accouchement should take place in spring, are apt to miscarry; and such as bring forth, have feeble and sickly children, so that they either die presently or are tender, feeble, and sickly, if they live. Such is the case with the women. The others are subject to dysenteries and dry ophthalmies, and some have catarrhs beginning in the head and descending to the lungs. Men of a phlegmatic temperament are likely to have dysenteries; and women, also, from the humidity of their nature, the phlegm descending downwards from the brain; those who are bilious, too, have dry ophthalmies from the heat and dryness of their flesh; the aged, too, have catarrhs from their flabbiness and melting of the veins, so that some of them die suddenly and some become paralytic on the right side or the left. For when, the winter being southerly and the body hot, the blood and veins are not properly constringed; a spring that is northerly, dry, and cold, having come on, the brain when it should have been expanded and purged, by the coryza and hoarseness is then constringed and contracted, so that the summer and the heat occurring suddenly, and a change supervening, these diseases fall out. And such cities as lie well to the sun and winds, and use good waters, feel these changes less, but such as use marshy and pooly waters, and lie well both as regards the winds and the sun, these all feel it more. And if the summer be dry, those diseases soon cease, but if rainy, they are protracted; and there is danger of any sore that there is becoming phagedenic from any cause; and lienteries and dropsies supervene at the conclusion of diseases; for the bowels are not readily dried up. And if the summer be rainy and southerly, and next the autumn, the winter must, of necessity, be sickly, and ardent fevers are likely to attack those that are phlegmatic, and more elderly than forty years, and pleurisies and peripneumonies those that are bilious. But if the summer is parched and northerly, but the autumn rainy and southerly, headache and sphacelus of the brain are likely to occur; and in addition hoarseness, coryza, coughs, and in some cases, consumption. But if the season is northerly and without water, there being no rain, neither after the Dogstar nor Arcturus; this state agrees best with those who are naturally phlegmatic, with those who are of a humid temperament, and with women; but it is most inimical to the bilious; for they become much parched up, and ophthalmies of a dry nature supervene, fevers both acute and chronic, and in some cases melancholy; for the most humid and watery part of the bile being consumed, the thickest and most acrid portion is left, and of the blood likewise, when these diseases came upon them. But all these are beneficial to the phlegmatic, for they are thereby dried up, and reach winter not oppressed with humors, but with them dried up.

11. Whoever studies and observes these things may be able to foresee most of the effects which will result from the changes of the seasons; and one ought to be particularly guarded during the greatest changes of the seasons, and neither willingly give medicines, nor apply the cautery to the belly, nor make incisions there until ten or more days be past. Now, the greatest and most dangerous are the two solstices, and especially the summer, and also the two equinoxes, but especially the autumnal. One ought also to be guarded about the rising of the stars, especially of the Dogstar, then of Arcturus, and then the setting of the Pleiades; for diseases are especially apt to prove critical in those days, and some prove fatal, some pass off, and all others change to another form and another constitution. So it is with regard to them.

12. I wish to show, respecting Asia and Europe, how, in all respects, they differ from one another, and concerning the figure of the inhabitants, for they are different, and do not at all resemble one another. To treat of all would be a long story, but I will tell you how I think it is with regard to the greatest and most marked differences. I say, then, that Asia differs very much from Europe as to the nature of all things, both With regard to the productions of the earth and the inhabitants, for everything is produced much more beautiful and large in Asia; the country is milder, and the dispositions of the inhabitants also are more gentle and affectionate. The cause of this is the temperature of the seasons, because it lies in the middle of the risings of the sun towards the east, and removed from the cold (and heat), for nothing tends to growth and mildness so much as when the climate has no predominant quality, but a general equality of temperature prevails. It is not everywhere the same with regard to Asia, but such parts of the country as lie intermediate between the heat and the cold, are the best supplied with fruits and trees, and have the most genial climate, and enjoy the purest waters, both celestial and terrestrial. For neither are they much burnt up by the heat, nor dried up by the drought and want of rain, nor do they suffer from the cold; since they are well watered from abundant showers and snow, and the fruits of the season, as might be supposed, grow in abundance, both such as are raised from seed that has been sown, and such plants as the earth produces of its own accord, the fruits of which the inhabitants make use of, training them from their wild state and transplanting them to a suitable soil; the cattle also which are reared there are vigorous, particularly prolific, and bring up young of the fairest description; the inhabitants too, are well fed, most beautiful in shape, of large stature, and differ little from one another either as to figure or size; and the country itself, both as regards its constitution and mildness of the seasons, may be said to bear a close resemblance to the spring. Manly courage, endurance of suffering, laborious enterprise, and high spirit, could not be produced in such a state of things either among the native inhabitants or those of a different country, for there pleasure necessarily reigns. For this reason, also, the forms of wild beasts there are much varied. Thus it is, as I think, with the Egyptians and Libyans.

13. But concerning those on the right hand of the summer risings of the sun as far as the Palus Maeotis (for this is the boundary of Europe and Asia), it is with them as follows: the inhabitants there differ far more from one another than those I have treated of above, owing to the differences of the seasons and the nature of the soil. But with regard to the country itself, matters are the same there as among all other men; for where the seasons undergo the greatest and most rapid changes, there the country is the wildest and most unequal; and you will find the greatest variety of mountains, forests, plains, and meadows; but where the seasons do not change much there the country is the most even; and, if one will consider it, so is it also with regard to the inhabitants; for the nature of some is like to a country covered with trees and well watered; of some, to a thin soil deficient in water; of others, to fenny and marshy places; and of some again, to a plain of bare and parched land. For the seasons which modify their natural frame of body are varied, and the greater the varieties of them the greater also will be the differences of their shapes.

14. I will pass over the smaller differences among the nations, but will now treat of such as are great either from nature, or custom; and, first, concerning the Macrocephali. There is no other race of men which have heads in the least resembling theirs. At first, usage was the principal cause of the length of their head, but now nature cooperates with usage. They think those the most noble who have the longest heads. It is thus with regard to the usage: immediately after the child is born, and while its head is still tender, they fashion it with their hands, and constrain it to assume a lengthened shape by applying bandages and other suitable contrivances whereby the spherical form of the head is destroyed, and it is made to increase in length. Thus, at first, usage operated, so that this constitution was the result of force: but, in the course of time, it was formed naturally; so that usage had nothing to do with it; for the semen comes from all parts of the body, sound from the sound parts, and unhealthy from the unhealthy parts. If, then, children with bald heads are born to parents with bald heads; and children with blue eyes to parents who have blue eyes; and if the children of parents having distorted eyes squint also for the most part; and if the same may be said of other forms of the body, what is to prevent it from happening that a child with a long head should be produced by a parent having a long head? But now these things do not happen as they did formerly, for the custom no longer prevails owing to their intercourse with other men. Thus it appears to me to be with regard to them.

15. As to the inhabitants of Phasis, their country is fenny, warm, humid, and wooded; copious and severe rains occur there at all seasons; and the life of the inhabitants is spent among the fens; for their dwellings are constructed of wood and reeds, and are erected amidst the waters; they seldom practice walking either to the city or the market, but sail about, up and down, in canoes constructed out of single trees, for there are many canals there. They drink the hot and stagnant waters, both when rendered putrid by the sun, and when swollen with rains. The Phasis itself is the most stagnant of all rivers, and runs the smoothest; all the fruits which spring there are unwholesome, feeble and imperfect growth, owing to the redundance of water, and on this account they do not ripen, for much vapor from the waters overspreads the country. For these reasons the Phasians have shapes different from those of all other men; for they are large in stature, and of a very gross habit of body, so that not a joint nor vein is visible; in color they are sallow, as if affected with jaundice. Of all men they have the roughest voices, from their breathing an atmosphere which is not clear, but misty and humid; they are naturally rather languid in supporting bodily fatigue. The seasons undergo but little change either as to heat or cold; their winds for the most part are southerly, with the exception of one peculiar to the country, which sometimes blows strong, is violent and hot, and is called by them the wind cenchron. The north wind scarcely reaches them, and when it does blow it is weak and gentle. Thus it is with regard to the different nature and shape of the inhabitants of Asia and Europe.

16. And with regard to the pusillanimity and cowardice of the inhabitants, the principal reason the Asiatics are more unwarlike and of gentler disposition than the Europeans is, the nature of the seasons, which do not undergo any great changes either to heat or cold, or the like; for there is neither excitement of the understanding nor any strong change of the body whereby the temper might be ruffled and they be roused to inconsiderate emotion and passion, rather than living as they do always in the state. It is changes of all kinds which arouse understanding of mankind, and do not allow them to get into a torpid condition. For these reasons, it appears to me, the Asiatic race is feeble, and further, owing to their laws; for monarchy prevails in the greater part of Asia, and where men are not their own masters nor independent, but are the slaves of others, it is not a matter of consideration with them how they may acquire military discipline, but how they may seem not to be warlike, for the dangers are not equally shared, since they must serve as soldiers, perhaps endure fatigue, and die for their masters, far from their children, their wives, and other friends; and whatever noble and manly actions they may perform lead only to the aggrandizement of their masters, whilst the fruits which they reap are dangers and death; and, in addition to all this, the lands of such persons must be laid waste by the enemy and want of culture. Thus, then, if any one be naturally warlike and courageous, his disposition will be changed by the institutions. As a strong proof of all this, such Greeks or barbarians in Asia as are not under a despotic form of government, but are independent, and enjoy the fruits of their own labors, are of all others the most warlike; for these encounter dangers on their own account, bear the prizes of their own valor, and in like manner endure the punishment of their own cowardice. And you will find the Asiatics differing from one another, for some are better and others more dastardly; of these differences, as I stated before, the changes of the seasons are the cause. Thus it is with Asia.

17. In Europe there is a Scythian race, called Sauromatae, which inhabits the confines of the Palus Maeotis, and is different from all other races. Their women mount on horseback, use the bow, and throw the javelin from their horses, and fight with their enemies as long as they are virgins; and they do not lay aside their virginity until they kill three of their enemies, nor have any connection with men until they perform the sacrifices according to law. Whoever takes to herself a husband, gives up riding on horseback unless the necessity of a general expedition obliges her. They have no right breast; for while still of a tender age their mothers heat strongly a copper instrument constructed for this very purpose, and apply it to the right breast, which is burnt up, and its development being arrested, all the strength and fullness are determined to the right shoulder and arm.

18. As the other Scythians have a peculiarity of shape, and do not resemble any other, the same observation applies to the Egyptians, only that the latter are oppressed by heat and the former by cold. What is called the Scythian desert is a prairie, rich in meadows, high-lying, and well watered; for the rivers which carry off the water from the plains are large. There live those Scythians which are called Nomades, because they have no houses, but live in wagons. The smallest of these wagons have four wheels, but some have six; they are covered in with felt, and they are constructed in the manner of houses, some having but a single apartment, and some three; they are proof against rain, snow, and winds. The wagons are drawn by yokes of oxen, some of two and others of three, and all without horns, for they have no horns, owing to the cold. In these wagons the women live, but the men are carried about on horses, and the sheep, oxen, and horses accompany them; and they remain on any spot as long as there is provender for their cattle, and when that fails they migrate to some other place. They eat boiled meat, and drink the milk of mares, and also eat hippace, which is cheese prepared from the milk of the mare. Such is their mode of life and their customs.

19. In respect of the seasons and figure of body, the Scythian race, like the Egyptian, have a uniformity of resemblance, different from all other nations; they are by no means prolific, and the wild beasts which are indigenous there are small in size and few in number, for the country lies under the Northern Bears, and the Rhiphaean mountains, whence the north wind blows;

the sun comes very near to them only when in the summer solstice, and warms them but for a short period, and not strongly;
and the winds blowing from the hot regions of the earth do not
reach them, or but seldom, and with little force; but the winds
from the north always blow, congealed, as they are, by the snow,
ice, and much water, for these never leave the mountains, which
are thereby rendered uninhabitable. A thick fog covers the plains
during the day, and amidst it they live, so that winter may be
said to be always present with them; or, if they have summer,
it is only for a few days, and the heat is not very strong. Their
plains are high-lying and naked, not crowned with mountains,
but extending upwards under the Northern Bears. The wild
beasts there are not large, but such as can be sheltered under-
ground; for the cold of winter and the barrenness of the country prevent their growth, and because they have no covert nor
shelter. The changes of the seasons, too, are not great nor violent,
for, in fact, they change gradually; and therefore their figures
resemble one another, as they all equally use the same food, and
the same clothing summer and winter, respiring a humid and
dense atmosphere, and drinking water from snow and ice; neither do they make any laborious exertions, for neither body nor
mind is capable of enduring fatigue when the changes of the
seasons are not great. For these reasons their shapes are gross
and fleshy, with ill-marked joints, of a humid temperament, and
deficient in tone: the internal cavities, and especially those of
the intestines, are full of humors; for the belly cannot possibly
be dry in such a country, with such a constitution and in such
a climate; but owing to their fat, and the absence of hairs from
their bodies, their shapes resemble one another, the males being
all alike, and so also with the women; for the seasons being of a
uniform temperature, no corruption or deterioration takes place

in the concretion of the semen, unless from some violent cause, or from disease.

20. I Will give you a strong proof of the humidity (laxity?) of their constitutions. You will find the greater part of the Scythians, and all the Nomades, with marks of the cautery on their shoulders, arms, wrists, breasts, hip-joints, and loins, and that for no other reason but the humidity and flabbiness of their constitution, for they can neither strain with their bows, nor launch the javelin from their shoulder owing to their humidity and atony: but when they are burnt, much of the humidity in their joints is dried up, and they become better braced, better fed, and their joints get into a more suitable condition. They are flabby and squat at first, because, as in Egypt, they are not swathed (?); and then they pay no attention to horsemanship, so that they may be adepts at it; and because of their sedentary mode of life; for the males, when they cannot be carried about on horseback, sit the most of their time in the wagon, and rarely practise walking, because of their frequent migrations and shiftings of situation; and as to the women, it is amazing how flabby and sluggish they are. The Scythian race are tawny from the cold, and not from the intense heat of the sun, for the whiteness of the skin is parched by the cold, and becomes tawny.

21. It is impossible that persons of such a constitution could be prolific, for, with the man, the sexual desires are not strong, owing to the laxity of his constitution, the softness and coldness of his belly, from all which causes it is little likely that a man should be given to venery; and besides, from being jaded by exercise on horseback, the men become weak in their desires. On the part of the men these are the causes; but on that of the women, they are embonpoint and humidity; for the womb cannot take in the semen, nor is the menstrual discharge such as it should be, but scanty and at too long intervals; and the mouth of the womb is shut up by fat and does not admit the semen; and, moreover, they themselves are indolent and fat, and their bellies cold and soft. From these causes the Scythian race is not prolific. Their female servants furnish a strong proof of this; for they no sooner have connection with a man than they prove with child, owing to their active course of life and the slenderness of body.

22. And, in addition to these, there are many eunuchs among the Scythians, who perform female work, and speak like women. Such persons are called effeminates. The inhabitants of the country attribute the cause of their impotence to a god, and venerate and worship such persons, every one dreading that the like might befall himself; but to me it appears that such affections are just as much divine as all others are, and that no one disease is either more divine or more human than another, but that all are alike divine, for that each has its own nature, and that no one arises without a natural cause. But I will explain how I think that the affection takes its rise. From continued exercise on horseback they are seized with chronic defluxions in their joints owing to their legs always hanging down below their horses; they afterwards become lame and stiff at the hip-joint, such of them, at least, as are severely attacked with it. They treat themselves in this way: when the disease is commencing, they open the vein behind either ear, and when the blood flows, sleep, from feebleness, seizes them, and afterwards they awaken, some in good health and others not. To me it appears that the semen is altered by this treatment, for there are veins behind the ears which, if cut, induce impotence; now, these veins would appear to me to be cut. Such persons afterwards, when they go in to women and cannot have connection with them, at first do not think much about it, but remain quiet; but when, after making the attempt two, three, or more times, they succeed no better, fancying they have committed some offence against the god whom they blame for the affection, they put on female attire, reproach themselves for effeminacy, play the part of women, and perform the same work as women do. This the rich among the Scythians endure, not the basest, but the most noble and powerful, owing to their riding on horseback; for the poor are less affected, as they do not ride on horses. And yet, if this disease had been more divine than the others, it ought not to have befallen the most noble and the richest of the Scythians alone, but all alike, or rather those who have little, as not being able to pay honors to the gods, if, indeed, they delight in being thus rewarded by men, and grant favors in return; for it is likely that the rich sacrifice more to the gods, and dedicate more votive offerings, inasmuch as they have wealth, and worship the gods; whereas the poor, from want, do less in this way, and, moreover, upbraid the gods for not giving them wealth, so that those who have few possessions were more likely to bear the punishments of these offences than the rich. But, as I formerly said, these affections are divine just as much as others, for each springs from a natural cause, and this disease arises among the Scythians from such a cause as I have stated. But it attacks other men in like manner, for whenever men ride much and very frequently on horseback, then many are affected with rheums in the joints, sciatica, and gout, and they are inept at venery. But these complaints befall the Scythians, and they are the most impotent of men for the aforesaid causes, and because they always wear breeches, and spend the most of their time on horseback, so as not to touch their privy parts with the hands, and from the cold and fatigue they forget the sexual desire, and do not make the attempt until after they have lost their virility. Thus it is with the race of the Scythians.

23. The other races in Europe differ from one another, both as to stature and shape, owing to the changes of the seasons, which are very great and frequent, and because the heat is strong, the winters severe, and there are frequent rains, and again protracted droughts, and winds, from which many and diversified changes are induced. These changes are likely to have an effect upon generation in the coagulation of the semen, as this process cannot be the same in summer as in winter, nor in rainy as in dry weather; wherefore, I think, that the figures of Europeans differ more than those of Asiatics; and they differ very much from one another as to stature in the same city; for vitiations of the semen occur in its coagulation more frequently during frequent changes of the seasons, than where they are alike and equable. And the same may be said of their dispositions, for the wild, and unsociable, and the passionate occur in such a constitution; for frequent excitement of the mind induces wildness, and extinguishes sociableness and mildness of disposition, and therefore I think the inhabitants of Europe more courageous than those of Asia; for a climate which is always the same induces indolence, but a changeable climate, laborious exertions both of body and mind; and from rest and indolence cowardice is engendered, and from laborious exertions and pains, courage. On this account the inhabitants of Europe are than the Asiatics, and also owing to their institutions, because they are not governed by kings like the latter, for where men are governed by kings there they must be very cowardly, as I have stated before; for their souls are enslaved, and they will not willingly, or readily undergo dangers in order to promote the power of another; but those that are free undertake dangers on their own account, and not for the sake of others; they court hazard and go out to meet it, for they themselves bear off the rewards of victory, and thus their institutions contribute not a little to their courage.

Such is the general character of Europe and Asia.

24. And there are in Europe other tribes, differing from one another in stature, shape, and courage: the differences are those I formerly mentioned, and will now explain more clearly. Such as inhabit a country which is mountainous, rugged, elevated, and well watered, and where the changes of the seasons are very great, are likely to have great variety of shapes among them, and to be naturally of an enterprising and warlike disposition; and such persons are apt to have no little of the savage and ferocious in their nature; but such as dwell in places which are low-lying, abounding in meadows and ill ventilated, and who have a larger proportion of hot than of cold winds, and who make use of warm waters—these are not likely to be of large stature nor well proportioned, but are of a broad make, fleshy, and have black hair; and they are rather of a dark than of a light complexion, and are less likely to be phlegmatic than bilious; courage and laborious enterprise are not naturally in them, but may be engendered in them by means of their institutions. And if there be rivers in the country which carry off the stagnant and rain water from it, these may be wholesome and clear; but if there be no rivers, but the inhabitants drink the waters of fountains, and such as are stagnant and marshy, they must necessarily have prominent bellies and enlarged spleens. But such as inhabit a high country, and one that is level, windy, and well-watered, will be large of stature, and like to one another; but their minds will be rather unmanly and gentle. Those who live on thin, ill-watered, and bare soils, and not well attempered in the changes of the seasons, in such a country they are likely to be in their persons rather hard and well braced, rather of a blond than a dark complexion, and in disposition and passions haughty and self-willed. For, where the changes of the seasons are most frequent, and where they differ most from one another, there you will find their forms, dispositions, and nature the most varied. These are the strongest of the natural causes of difference, and next the country in which one lives, and the waters; for, in general, you will find the forms and dispositions of mankind to correspond with the nature of the country; for where the land is fertile, soft, and well-watered, and supplied with waters from very elevated situations, so as to be hot in summer and cold in winter, and where the seasons are fine, there the men are fleshy, have ill-formed joints, and are of a humid temperament; they are not disposed to endure labor, and, for the most part, are base in spirit; indolence and sluggishness are visible in them, and to the arts they are dull, and not clever nor acute. When the country is bare, not fenced, and rugged, blasted by the winter and scorched by the sun, there you may see the hardy, hardy, slender, with well-shaped joints, well-braced, and shaggy; sharp, industry and vigilance accompany such a constitution; in morals and passions they are haughty and opinionative, inclining rather to the fierce than to the mild; and you will find them acute and ingenious as regards the arts, and excelling in military affairs; and likewise all the other productions of the earth corresponding to the earth itself. Thus it is with regard to the most opposite natures and shapes; drawing conclusions from them, you may judge of the rest without any risk of error.

OF THE EPIDEMICS

BOOK I.

Sect. I. First Constitution

1. IN THASUS, about the autumn equinox, and under the Pleiades, the rains were abundant, constant, and soft, with southerly winds; the winter southerly, the northerly winds faint, droughts; on the whole, the winter having the character of spring. The spring was southerly, cool, rains small in quantity. Summer, for the most part, cloudy, no rain, the Etesian winds, rare and small, blew in an irregular manner. The whole constitution of the season being thus inclined to the southerly, and with droughts early in the spring, from the preceding opposite and northerly state, ardent fevers occurred in a few instances, and these very mild, being rarely attended with hemorrhage, and never proving fatal. Swellings appeared about the ears, in many on either side, and in the greatest number on both sides, being unaccompanied by fever so as not to confine the patient to bed; in all cases they disappeared without giving trouble, neither did any of them come to suppuration, as is common in swellings from other causes. They were of a lax, large, diffused character, without inflammation or pain, and they went away without any critical sign. They seized children, adults, and mostly those who were engaged in the exercises of the palestra and gymnasium, but seldom attacked women. Many had dry coughs without expectoration, and accompanied with hoarseness of voice. In some instances earlier, and in others later, inflammations with pain seized sometimes one of the testicles, and sometimes both; some of these cases were accompanied with fever and some not; the greater part of these were attended with much suffering. In other respects they were free of disease, so as not to require medical assistance.

2. Early in the beginning of spring, and through the summer, and towards winter, many of those who had been long gradually declining, took to bed with symptoms of phthisis; in many cases formerly of a doubtful character the disease then became confirmed; in these the constitution inclined to the phthisical. Many, and, in fact, the most of them, died; and of those confined to bed, I do not know if a single individual survived for any considerable time; they died more suddenly than is common in such cases. But other diseases, of a protracted character, and attended with fever, were well supported, and did not prove fatal: of these we will give a description afterwards. Consumption was the most considerable of the diseases which then prevailed, and the only one which proved fatal to many persons. Most of them were affected by these diseases in the following manner: fevers accompanied with rigors, of the continual type, acute, having no complete intermissions, but of the form of the semi-tertians, being milder the one day, and the next having an exacerbation, and increasing in violence; constant sweats, but not diffused over the whole body; extremities very cold, and warmed with difficulty; bowels disordered, with bilious, scanty, unmixed, thin, pungent, and frequent dejections. The urine was thin, colorless, unconcocted, or thick, with a deficient sediment, not settling favorably, but casting down a crude and unseasonable sediment. Sputa small, dense, concocted, but brought up rarely and with difficulty; and in those who encountered the most violent symptoms there was no concoction at all, but they continued throughout spitting crude matters. Their fauces, in most of them, were painful from first to last, having redness with inflammation; defluxions thin, small and acrid; they were soon wasted and became worse, having no appetite for any kind of food throughout; no thirst; most persons delirious when near death. So much concerning the phthisical affections.

3. In the course of the summer and autumn many fevers of the continual type, but not violent; they attacked persons who had been long indisposed, but who were otherwise not in an uncomfortable state. In most cases the bowels were disordered in a very moderate degree, and they did not suffer thereby in any manner worth mentioning; the urine was generally well colored, clear, thin, and after a time becoming concocted near the crisis. They had not much cough, nor it troublesome; they were not in appetite, for it was necessary to give them food (on the whole, persons laboring under phthisis were not affected in the usual manner). They were affected with fevers, rigors, and deficient sweats, with varied and irregular paroxysms, in general not inter-mitting, but having exacerbations in the tertian form. The earliest crisis which occurred was about the twentieth day, in most about the fortieth, and in many about the eightieth. But there were cases in which it did not leave them thus at all, but in an irregular manner, and without any crisis; in most of these the fevers, after a brief interval, relapsed again; and from these relapses they came to a crisis in the same periods; but in many they were prolonged so that the disease was not gone at the approach of winter. Of all those which are described under this constitution, the phthisical diseases alone were of a fatal character; for in all the others the patients bore up well, and did not die of the other fevers.

Sect. II. Second Constitution

1. In Thasus, early in autumn, the winter suddenly set in rainy before the usual time, with much northerly and southerly winds. These things all continued so during the season of the Pleiades, and until their setting. The winter was northerly, the rains frequent, in torrents, and large, with snow, but with a frequent mixture of fair weather. These things were all so, but the setting in of the cold was not much out of season. After the winter solstice, and at the time when the zephyr usually begins to blow, severe winterly storms out of season, with much northerly wind, snow, continued and copious rains; the sky tempestuous and clouded; these things were protracted, and did not remit until the equinox. The spring was cold, northerly, rainy, and clouded; the summer was not very sultry, the Etesian winds blew constant, but quickly afterwards, about the rising of Arcturus, there were again many rains with north winds. The whole season being wet, cold, and northerly, people were, for the most part, healthy during winter; but early in the spring very many, indeed, the greater part, were valetudinary. At first ophthalmies set in, with rheums, pains, unconcocted discharges, small concretions, generally breaking with difficulty, in most instances they relapsed, and they did not cease until late in autumn. During summer and autumn there were dysenteric affections, attacks of tenesmus and lientery, bilious diarrhoea, with thin, copious, undigested, and acrid dejections, and sometimes with watery stools; many had copious defluxions, with pain, of a bilious, watery, slimy, purulent nature, attended with strangury, not connected with disease of the kidneys, but one complaint succeeding the other; vomitings of bile, phlegm, and undigested food, sweats, in all cases a reduncance of humors. In many instances these complaints were unattended with fever, and did not prevent the patients from walking about, but some cases were febrile, as will be described. In some all those described below occurred with pain. During autumn, and at the commencement of winter, there were phthisical complaints, continual fevers; and, in a few cases, ardent; some diurnal, others nocturnal, semi-tertians, true tertians, quartans, irregular fevers.

2. All these fevers described attacked great numbers. All these fevers attacked the smallest numbers, and the patients suffered the least from them, for there were no hemorrhages, except a few and to a small amount, nor was there delirium; all the other complaints were slight; in these the crises were regular, in most instances, with the intermittents, in seventeen days; and I know no instance of a person dying of causus, nor becoming phrenitic. The tertians were more numerous than the ardent fevers, and attended with more pain; but these all had four periods in regular succession from the first attack, and they had a complete crisis in seven, without a relapse in any instance. The quartans attacked many at first, in the form of regular quartans, but in no few cases a transition from other fevers and diseases into quartans took place; they were protracted, as is wont with them, indeed, more so than usual. Quotidian, nocturnal, and wandering fevers attacked many persons, some of whom continued to keep up, and others were confined to bed. In most instances these fevers were prolonged under the Pleiades and till winter. Many persons, and more especially children, had convulsions from the commencement; and they had fever, and the convulsions supervened upon the fevers; in most cases they were protracted, but free from danger, unless in those who were in a deadly state from other complaints. Those fevers which were continual in the main, and with no intermissions, but having exacerbations in the

tertian form, there being remissions the one day and exacerbations the next, were the most violent of all those which occurred at that time, and the most protracted, and occurring with the greatest pains, beginning mildly, always on the whole increasing, and being exacerbated, and always turning worse, having small remissions, and after an abatement having more violent paroxysms, and growing worse, for the most part, on the critical days. Rigors, in all cases, took place in an irregular and uncertain manner, very rare and weak in them, but greater in all other fevers; frequent sweats, but most seldom in them, bringing no alleviation, but, on the contrary, doing mischief. Much cold of the extremities in them, and these were warmed with difficulty. Insomnolency, for the most part, especially in these fevers, and again a disposition to coma. The bowels, in all diseases, were disordered, and in a bad state, but worst of all in these. The urine, in most of them, was either thin and crude, yellow, and after a time with slight symptoms of concoction in a critical form, or having the proper thickness, but muddy, and neither settling nor subsiding; or having small and bad, and crude sediments; these being the worst of all. Coughs attended these fevers, but I cannot state that any harm or good ever resulted from the cough.

3. The most of these were protracted and troublesome, went on in a very disorderly and irregular form, and, for the most part, did in a crisis, either in the fatal cases or in the others; for if it left some of them for a season it soon returned again. In a few instances the lever terminated with a crisis; in the earliest of these about the eightieth day, and some of these relapsed, so that most of them were not free from the fever during the winter; but the fever left most of them without a crisis, and these things happened alike to those who recovered and to those who did not. There being much want of crisis and much variety as to these diseases, the greatest and worst symptom attended the most of them, namely, a loathing of all articles of food, more especially with those who had otherwise fatal symptoms; but they were not unseasonably thirsty in such fevers. After a length of time, with much suffering and great wasting, abscesses were formed in these cases, either unusually large, so that the patients could not support them, or unusually small, so that they did no good, but soon relapsed and speedily got worse. The diseases which attacked them were in the form of dysenteries, tenesmus, lientery, and fluxes; but, in some cases, there were dropsies, with or without these complaints. Whatever attacked them violently speedily cut them off, or again, did them no good. Small rashes, and not corresponding to the violence of the disease, and quickly disappearing, or swellings occurred about the ears, which were not resolved, and brought on no crisis. In some they were determined to the joints, and especially to the hip-joint, terminating critically with a few, and quickly again increasing to its original habit.

4. People died of all these diseases, but mostly of these fevers, and notably infants just weaned, and older children, until eight or ten years of age, and those before puberty. These things occurred to those affected with the complaints described above, and to many persons at first without them. The only favorable symptom, and the greatest of those which occurred, and what saved most of those who were in the greatest dangers, was the conversion of it to a strangury, and when, in addition to this, abscesses were formed. The strangury attacked, most especially, persons of the ages I have mentioned, but it also occurred in many others, both of those who were not confined to bed and those who were. There was a speedy and great change in all these cases. For the bowels, if they happened previously to have watery discharges of a bad character, became regular, they got an appetite for food, and the fevers were mild afterwards. But, with regard to the strangury itself, the symptoms were protracted and painful. Their urine was copious, thick, of various characters, red, mixed with pus, and was passed with pain. These all recovered, and I did not see a single instance of death among them.

5. With regard to the dangers of these cases, one must always attend to the seasonable concoction of all the evacuations, and to the favorable and critical abscesses. The concoctions indicate a speedy crisis and recovery of health; crude and undigested evacuations, and those which are converted into bad abscesses, indicate either want of crisis, or pains, or prolongation of the disease, or death, or relapses; which of these it is to be must be determined from other circumstances. The physician must be able to tell the antecedents, know the present, and foretell the future—must mediate these things, and have two special objects in view with regard to disease, namely, to do good or to do no harm. The art consists in three things—the disease, the patient, and the physician. The physician is the servant of the art, and the patient must combat the disease along with the physician.

6. Pains about the head and neck, and heaviness of the same along with pain, occur either without fevers or in fevers. Convulsions occurring in persons attacked with frenzy, and having vomitings of verdigris-green bile, in some cases quickly prove fatal. In ardent fevers, and in those other fevers in which there is pain of the neck, heaviness of the temples, mistiness about the eyes, and distention about the hypochondriac region, not unattended with pain, hemorrhage from the nose takes place, but those who have heaviness of the whole head, cardialgia and nausea, vomit bilious and pituitous matters; children, in such affections, are generally attacked with convulsions, and women have these and also pains of the uterus; whereas, in elder persons, and those in whom the heat is already more subdued, these cases end in paralysis, mania, and loss of sight.

Third Constitution

7. In Thasus, a little before and during the season of Arcturus, there were frequent and great rains, with northerly winds. About the equinox, and till the setting of the Pleiades, there were a few southerly rains: the winter northerly and parched, cold, with great winds and snow. Great storms about the equinox, the spring northerly, dryness, rains few and cold. About the summer solstice, scanty rains, and great cold until near the season of the Dog-star. After the Dog-days, until the season of Arcturus, the summer hot, great droughts, not in intervals, but continued and severe: no rain; the Etesian winds blew; about the season of Arcturus southerly rains until the equinox.

8. In this state of things, during winter, paraplegia set in, and attacked many, and some died speedily; and otherwise the disease prevailed much in an epidemical form, but persons remained free from all other diseases. Early in the spring, ardent fevers commenced and continued through the summer until the equinox. Those then that were attacked immediately after the commencement of the spring and summer, for the most part recovered, and but few of them died. But when the autumn and the rains had set in, they were of a fatal character, and the greater part then died. When in these attacks of ardent fevers there was a proper and copious hemorrhage from the nose, they were generally saved by it, and I do not know a single person who had a proper hemorrhage who died in this constitution. Philiscus, Epaminon, and Silenus, indeed, who had a trifling epistaxis on the fourth and fifth day, died. Most of those taken with had a

rigor about the time of the crisis, and notably those who had no hemorrhage; these had also rigor associated.

9. Some were attacked with jaundice on the sixth day, but these were benefited either by an urinary purgation, or a disorder of the bowels, or a copious hemorrhage, as in the case of Heraclides, who was lodged with Aristocydes: this person, though he had the hemorrhage from the nose, the purgation by the bladder, and disorder of the bowels, experienced a favorable crisis on the twentieth day, not like the servant of Phanagoras, who had none of these symptoms, and died. The hemorrhages attacked most persons, but especially young persons and those in the prime of life, and the greater part of those who had not the hemorrhage died: elderly persons had jaundice or disorder of the bowels, such as Bion, who was lodged with Silenus. Dysenteries were epidemical during the summer, and some of those cases in which the hemorrhage occurred, terminated in dysentery, as happened to the slave of Eraton, and to Mullus, who had a copious hemorrhage, which settled down into dysentery, and they recovered. This humor was redundant in many cases, since in those who had not the hemorrhage about the crisis, but the risings about the ears disappeared, after their disappearance there was a sense of weight in the left flank extending to the extremity of the hip, and pain setting in after the crisis, with a discharge of thin urine; they began to have small hemorrhages about the twenty-fourth day, and the swelling was converted into the hemorrhage. In the case of Antiphon, the son of Critobulus' son, the fever ceased and came to a crisis about the fortieth day.

10. Many women were seized, but fewer than of the men, and there were fewer deaths among them. But most of them had difficult parturition, and after labor they were taken ill, and these most especially died, as, for example, the daughter of Telebolus died on the sixth day after delivery. Most females had the menstrual discharge during the fever, and many girls had it then for the first time: in certain individuals both the hemorrhage from the nose and the menses appeared; thus, in the case of the virgin daughter of Daetharses, the menses then took place for the first time, and she had also a copinous hemorrhage from the nose, and I knew no instance of any one dying when one or other of these took place properly. But all those in the pregnant state that were attacked had abortions, as far as I observed. The urine in most cases was of the proper color, but thin, and having scanty sediments: in most the bowels were disordered with thin and bilious dejections; and many, after passing through the other crises, terminated in dysenteries, as happened to Xenophanes and Critias. The urine was watery, copious, clear, and thin; and even after the crises, when the sediment was natural, and all the other critical symptoms were favorable, as I recollect having happened to Bion, who was lodged in the house of Silenus, and Critias, who lived with Xenophanes, the slave of Areton, and the wife of Mnesistratus. But afterwards all these were attacked with dysentery. It would be worth while to inquire whether the watery urine was the cause of this. About the season of Arcturus many had the crisis on the eleventh day, and in them the regular relapses did not take place, but they became comatose about this time, especially children; but there were fewest deaths of all among them.

11. About the equinox, and until the season of the Pleiades, and at the approach of winter, many ardent fevers set in; but great numbers at that season were seized with phrenitis, and many died; a few cases also occurred during the summer. These then made their attack at the commencement of ardent fevers, which were attended with fatal symptoms; for immediately upon

their setting in, there were acute fever and small rigors, insomnolency, aberration, thirst, nausea, insignificant sweats about the forehead and clavicles, but no general perspiration; they had much delirious talking, fears, despondency, great coldness of the extremities, in the feet, but more especially in their hands: the paroxysms were on the even days; and in most cases, on the fourth day, the most violent pains set in, with sweats, generally coldish, and the extremities could not be warmed, but were livid and rather cold, and they had then no thirst; in them the urine was black, scanty, thin, and the bowels were constipated; there was an hemorrhage from the nose in no case in which these symptoms occurred, but merely a trifling epistaxis; and none of them had a relapse, but they died on the sixth day with sweats. In the phrenitic cases, all the symptoms which have been described did not occur, but in them the disease mostly came to a crisis on the eleventh day, and in some on the twentieth. In those cases in which the phrenitis did not begin immediately, but about the third or fourth day, the disease was moderate at the commencement, but assumed a violent character about the seventh day. There was a great number of diseases, and of those affected, they who died were principally infants, young persons, adults having smooth bodies, white skins, straight and black hair, dark eyes, those living recklessly and luxuriously; persons with shrill, or rough voices, who stammered and were passionate, and women more especially died from this form. In this constitution, four symptoms in particular proved salutary; either a hemorrhage from the nose, or a copious discharge by the bladder of urine, having an abundant and proper sediment, or a bilious disorder of the bowels at the proper time, or an attack of dysentery. And in many cases it happened, that the crisis did not take place by any one of the symptoms which have been mentioned, but the patient passed through most of them, and appeared to be in an uncomfortable way, and yet all who were attacked with these symptoms recovered. All the symptoms which I have described occurred also to women and girls; and whoever of them had any of these symptoms in a favorable manner, or the menses appeared abundantly, were saved thereby, and had a crisis, so that I do not know a single female who had any of these favorably that died. But the daughter of Philo, who had a copious hemorrhage from the nose, and took supper unseasonably on the seventh day, died. In those cases of acute, and more especially of ardent fevers, in which there is an involuntary discharge of tears, you may expect a nasal hemorrhage unless the other symptoms be of a fatal type, for in those of a bad description, they do not indicate a hemorrhage, but death.

12. Swellings about the ears, with pain in fevers, sometimes when the fever went off critically, neither subsided nor were converted into pus; in these cases a bilious diarrhoea, or dysentery, or thick urine having a sediment, carried off the disease, as happened to Hermippus of Clazomenae. The circumstances relating to crises, as far as we can recognize them, were so far similar and so far dissimilar. Thus two brothers became ill at the same hour (they were brothers of Epigenes, and lodged near the theatre), of these the elder had a crisis on the sixth day, and the younger on the seventh, and both had a relapse at the same hour; it then left them for five days, and from the return of the fever both had a crisis together on the seventeenth day. Most had a crisis on the sixth day; it then left them for six days, and from the relapse there was a crisis on the fifth day. But those who had a crisis on the seventh day, had an intermission for seven days; and the crisis took place on the third day after the relapse. Those who had a crisis on the sixth day, after an interval of six days were seized again on the third, and having left them for one day, the fever attacked them again on the next and came to a crisis, as happened to Evagon the son of Daetharses. Those in whom the crisis happened on the sixth day, had an intermission of seven days, and from the relapse there was a crisis on the fourth, as happened to the daughter of Aglaidas. The greater part of those who were taken ill under this constitution of things, were affected in this manner, and I did not know a single case of recovery, in which there was not a relapse agreeably to the stated order of relapses; and all those recovered in which the relapses took place according to this form: nor did I know a single instance of those who then passed through the disease in this manner who had another relapse.

13. In these diseases death generally happened on the sixth day, as with Epaminondas, Silenus, and Philiscus the son of Antagoras. Those who had parotid swellings experienced a crisis on the twentieth day, but in all these cases the disease went off without coming to a suppuration, and was turned upon the bladder. But in Cratistonax, who lived by the temple of Hercules, and in the maid servant of Scymnus the fuller, it turned to a suppuration, and they died. Those who had a crisis on the seventh day, had an intermission of nine days, and a relapse which came to a crisis on the fourth day from the return of the fever, as was the case with Pantacles, who resided close by the temple of Bacchus. Those who had a crisis on the seventh day, after an interval of six days had a relapse, from which they had a crisis on the seventh day, as happened to Phanocritus, who was lodged with Gnathon the fuller. During the winter, about the winter solstices, and until the equinox, the ardent fevers and frenzies prevailed, and many died. The crisis, however, changed, and happened to the greater number on the fifth day from the commencement, left them for four days and relapsed; and after the return, there was a crisis on the fifth day, making in all fourteen days. The crisis took place thus in the case of most children, also in elder persons. Some had a crisis on the eleventh day, a relapse on the fourteenth, a complete crisis on the twentieth; but certain persons, who had a rigor about the twentieth, had a crisis on the fortieth. The greater part had a rigor along with the original crisis, and these had also a rigor about the crisis in the relapse. There were fewest cases of rigor in the spring, more in summer, still more in autumn, but by far the most in winter; then hemorrhages ceased.

Sect. III

1. With regard to diseases, the circumstances from which we form a judgment of them are,—by attending to the general nature of all, and the peculiar nature of each individual,—to the disease, the patient, and the applications,—to the person who applies them, as that makes a difference for better or for worse,—to the whole constitution of the season, and particularly to the state of the heavens, and the nature of each country;— to the patient's habits, regimen, and pursuits;—to his conversation, manners, taciturnity, thoughts, sleep, or absence of sleep, and sometimes his dreams, what and when they occur;—to his picking and scratching;—to his tears;—to the alvine discharges, urine, sputa, and vomitings; and to the changes of diseases from the one into the other;—to the deposits, whether of a deadly or critical character;—to the sweat, coldness, rigor, cough, sneezing, hiccup, respiration, eructation, flatulence, whether passed silently or with a noise;—to hemorrhages and hemorrhoids;—from these, and their consequences, we must form our judgment.

2. Fevers are,—the continual, some of which hold during the day and have a remission at night, and others hold a remission

during the day; semi-tertians, tertians, quartans, quintans, septans, nonans. The most acute, strongest, most dangerous, and fatal
diseases, occur in the continual fever. The least dangerous of all,
and the mildest and most protracted, is the quartan, for it is not
only such from itself, but it also carries off other great diseases.
In what is called the semi-tertian, other acute diseases are apt to
occur, and it is the most fatal of all others, and moreover phthisical persons, and those laboring under other protracted diseases,
are apt to be attacked by it. The nocturnal fever is not very fatal,
but protracted; the diurnal is still more protracted, and in some
cases passes into phthisis. The septan is protracted, but not fatal;
the nonan more protracted, and not fatal. The true tertian comes
quickly to a crisis, and is not fatal; but the quintan is the worst
of all, for it proves fatal when it precedes an attack of phthisis,
and when it supervenes on persons who are already consumptive. There are peculiar modes, and constitutions, and paroxysms,
in every one of these fevers; for example,—the continual, in
some cases at the very commencement, grows, as it were, and
attains its full strength, and rises to its most dangerous pitch, but
is diminished about and at the crisis; in others it begins gentle
and suppressed, but gains ground and is exacerbated every day,
and bursts forth with all its heat about and at the crisis; while
in others, again, it commences mildly, increases, and is exacerbated until it reaches its acme, and then remits until at and
about the crisis. These varieties occur in every fever, and in every
disease. From these observations one must regulate the regimen
accordingly. There are many other important symptoms allied to
these, part of which have been already noticed, and part will be
described afterwards, from a consideration of which one may
judge, and decided in each case, whether the disease be acute,
acute, and whether it will end in death or recovery; or whether it

will be protracted, and will end in death or recovery; and in what cases food is to be given, and in what not; and when and to what amount, and what particular kind of food is to be administered.

3. Those diseases which have their paroxysms on even days have their crises on even days; and those which have their paroxysms on uneven days have their crises on uneven days. The first period of those which have the crisis on even days, is the 4th, 6th, 8th, 10th, 14th, 20th, 30th, 40th, 60th, 80th, 100th; and the first period of those which have their crises on uneven days, is the 1st, 3d, 5th, 7th, 9th, 11th, 17th, 21th, 27th, 31st. It should be known, that if the crisis take place on any other day than on those described, it indicates that there will be a relapse, which may prove fatal. But one ought to pay attention, and know in these seasons what crises will lead to recovery and what to death, or to changes for the better or the worse. Irregular fevers, quartans, quintans, septans, and nonans should be studied, in order to find out in what periods their crises take place.

Fourteen Cases of Disease

CASE I. Philiscus, who lived by the Wall, took to bed on the first day of acute fever; he sweated; towards night was uneasy. On the second day all the symptoms were exacerbated; late in the evening had a proper stool from a small clyster; the night quiet. On the third day, early in the morning and until noon, he appeared to be free from fever; towards evening, acute fever, with sweating, thirst, tongue parched; passed black urine; night uncomfortable, no sleep; he was delirious on all subjects. On the fourth, all the symptoms exacerbated, urine black; night more comfortable, urine of a better color. On the fifth, about mid-day, had a slight trickling of pure blood from the nose; urine varied in character, having floating in it round bodies, resembling semen, and scattered, but which did not fall to the bottom; a suppository having been applied, some scanty flatulent matters were passed; night uncomfortable, little sleep, talking incoherently; extremities altogether cold, and could not be warmed; urine, black; slept a little towards day; loss of speech, cold sweats; extremities livid; about the middle of the sixth day he died. The respiration throughout, like that of a person recollecting himself, was rare, and large, and spleen was swelled upon in a round tumor, the sweats cold throughout, the paroxysms on the even days.

CASE II.   Silenus lived on the Broad-way, near the house of Evalcidas. From fatigue, drinking, and unseasonable exercises, he was seized with fever. He began with having pain in the loins; he had heaviness of the head, and there was stiffness of the neck. On the first day the alvine discharges were bilious, unmixed, frothy, high colored, and copious; urine black, having a black sediment; he was thirsty, tongue dry; no sleep at night. On the second, acute fever, stools more copious, thinner, frothy; urine black, an uncomfortable night, slight delirium. On the third, all the symptoms exacerbated; an oblong distention, of a softish nature, from both sides of the hypochondrium to the navel; stools thin, and darkish; urine muddy, and darkish; no sleep at night; much talking, laughter, singing, he could not restrain himself. On the fourth, in the same state. On the fifth, stools bilious, unmixed, smooth, greasy; urine thin, and transparent; slight absence of delirium. On the sixth, slight perspiration about the head; extremities cold and livid; much tossing about; no passage from the bowels, urine suppressed, acute fever. On the seventh, loss of speech; extremities could no longer be kept warm; no discharge of urine. On the eighth, a cold sweat all over; red rashes with sweat, of a round figure, small, like vari, persistent, not subsiding; by means of a slight stimulus, a copious discharge from the bowels, of a thin and undigested character, with pain; urine acrid, and passed with pain; extremities slightly heated; sleep slight, and comatose; speechless; urine thin, and transparent. On the ninth, in the same state. On the tenth, no drink taken; comatose, sleep slight; alvine discharges the same; urine abundant, and thickish; when allowed to stand, the sediment farinaceous and white; extremities again cold. On the eleventh, he died. At the commencement, and throughout, the respiration was slow and large; there was a constant throbbing in the hypochondrium; his age was about twenty.

CASE III. Herophon was seized with an acute fever; alvine discharges at first were scanty, and attended with tenesmus; but afterwards they were passed of a thin, bilious character, and frequent; there was no sleep; urine black, and thin. On the fifth, in the morning, deafness; all the symptoms exacerbated; spleen swollen; distention of the hypochondrium; alvine discharges scanty, and black; he became delirious. On the sixth, delirious; at night, sweating, coldness; the delirium continued. On the seventh, he became cold, thirsty, was disordered in mind; at night recovered his senses; slept. On the eighth, was feverish; the spleen diminished in size; quite collected; had pain at first about the groin, on the same side as the spleen; had pains in both legs; night comfortable; urine better colored, had a scanty sediment. On the ninth, sweated; the crisis took place; fever remitted. On the fifth day afterwards, fever relapsed, spleen immediately became swollen; acute fever; deafness again. On the third day after the relapse, the spleen diminished; deafness less; legs painful; sweated during the night; crisis took place on the seventeenth day; had no disorder of the senses during the relapse.

CASE IV. In Thasus, the wife of Philinus, having been delivered of a daughter, the discharge being natural, and other matters going on mildly, on the fourteenth day after delivery was seized with fever, attended with rigor; was pained at first in the cardiac region of the stomach and right hypochondrium; pain in the genital organs; lochial discharge ceased. Upon the application of a pessary all these symptoms were alleviated; pains of the head, neck, and loins remained; no sleep; extremities cold; thirst; bowels in a hot state; stools scanty; urine thin, and colorless at first. On the sixth, towards night, senses much disordered, but again were restored. On the seventh, thirsty; the evacuations bilious, and high colored. On the eighth, had a rigor; acute fever; much spasm, with pain; talked much, incoherently; upon the application of a suppository, rose to stool, and passed copious dejections, with a bilious flux; no sleep. On the ninth, spasms. On the tenth, slightly recollected. On the eleventh, slept; had perfect recollection, but again immediately wandered; passed a large quantity of urine with spasms, (the attendants seldom putting her in mind), it was thick, white, like urine which has been shaken after it has stood for a considerable time until it has subsided, but it had no sediment; in color and consistence, the urine resembled that of cattle, as far as I observed. About the fourteenth day, startings over the whole body; talked much; slightly collected, but presently became again delirious. About the seventeenth day became speechless, on the twentieth died.

CASE V. The wife of Epicrates, who was lodged at the house of Archigetes, being near the term of delivery, was seized with a violent rigor, and, as was said, she did not become heated; next day the same. On the third, she was delivered of a daughter, and everything went on properly. On the day following her delivery, she was seized with acute fever, pain in the cardiac region of the stomach, and in the genital parts. Having had a suppository, was in so far relieved; pain in the head, neck, and loins; no sleep;

alvine discharges scanty, bilious, thin, and unmixed; urine thin, and blackish. Towards the night of the sixth day from the time she was seized with the fever, became delirious. On the seventh, all the symptoms exacerbated; insomnolency, delirium, thirst; stools bilious, and high colored. On the eighth, had a rigor; slept more. On the ninth, the same. On the tenth, her limbs painfully affected; pain again of the cardiac region of the stomach; heaviness of the head; no delirium; slept more; bowels constipated. On the eleventh, passed urine of a better color, and having an abundant sediment; felt lighter. On the fourteenth had a rigor; acute fever. On the fifteenth, had a copious vomiting of bilious and yellow matters; sweated; fever gone; at night acute fever; urine thick, sediment white. On the seventeenth, an exacerbation; night uncomfortable; no sleep; delirium. On the eighteenth, thirsty; tongue parched; no sleep; much delirium; legs painfully affected. About the twentieth, in the morning, had as light rigor; was comatose; slept tranquilly; had slight vomiting of bilious and black matters; towards night deafness. About the twenty-first, weight generally in the left side, with pain; slight urine thick, muddy, and reddish; when allowed to stand, had no sediment; in other respects felt lighter; fever not gone; fauces painful from the commencement, and red; uvula retracted; defluxion remained acrid, pungent, and saltish throughout. About the twenty-seventh, free of fever; sediment in the urine; pain in the side. About the thirty-first, was attacked with fever, bilious diarrhea; slight bilious vomiting on the fortieth. Had a complete crisis, and was freed from the fever on the eightieth day.

CASE VI. Cleonactides, who was lodged above the Temple of Hercules, was seized with a fever in an irregular form; was pained in the head and left side from the commencement, and had other pains resembling those produced by fatigue; paroxysms of the fevers inconstant and irregular; occasional sweats; the paroxysms generally attacked on the critical days. About the twenty-fourth was cold in the extremities of the hands, vomitings bilious, yellow, and frequent, soon turning to a ver-digris-green color; general relief. About the thirtieth, began to have hemorrhage from both nostrils, and this continued in an irregular manner until near the crisis; did not loathe food, and had no thirst throughout, nor was troubled with insomnolency; urine thin, and not devoid of color. When about the thirtieth day, passed reddish urine, having a copious red sediment; was relieved, but afterwards the characters of the urine varied, some-times having sediment, and sometimes not. On the sixtieth, the sediment in the urine copious, white, and smooth; all the symptoms ameliorated; intermission of the fever; urine thin, and well colored. On the seventieth, fever gone for ten days. On the eightieth had a rigor, was seized with acute fever, sweated much; a red, smooth sediment in the urine; and a perfect crisis.

CASE VII. Meton was seized with fever; there was a painful weight in the loins. Next day, after drinking water pretty copi-ously, had proper evacuations from the bowels. On the third, heaviness of the head, stools thin, bilious, and reddish. On the fourth, all the symptoms exacerbated; had twice a scanty trickling of blood from the right nostril; passed an uncomfortable night; alvine discharges like those on the third day; urine darkish, had a darkish cloud floating in it, of a scattered form, which did not subside. On the fifth, a copious hemorrhage of pure blood from the left he sweated, and had a crisis. After the fever restless, and had some delirium; urine thin, and darkish; had an affusion of warm water on the head; slept and recovered his senses. In this case there was no relapse, but there were frequent hemorrhages after the crisis.

CASE VIII. Erasinus, who lived near the Canal of Bootes, was seized with fever after supper; passed the night in an agitated state. During the first day quiet, but in pain at night. On the second, symptoms all exacerbated; at night delirious. On the third, was in a painful condition; great incoherence. On the fourth, in a most uncomfortable state; had no sound sleep at night, but dreaming and talking; then all the appearances worse, of a formidable and alarming character; fear, impatience. On the morning of the fifth, was composed, and quite coherent, but long before noon was furiously mad, so that he could not constrain himself; extremities cold, and somewhat livid; urine without sediment; died about sunset. The fever in this case was accompanied by sweats throughout; the sweats throughout; the hypochondria were in a state of meteorism, with distention and pain; the urine was black, has round substances floating in it, which did not subside; the alvine evacuations were not stopped; thirst throughout not great; much spasms with sweats about the time of death.

CASE IX. Criton, in Thasus, while still on foot, and going about, was seized with a violent pain in the great toe; he took to bed the same day, had rigors and nausea, recovered his heat slightly, at night was delirious. On the second, swelling of the whole foot, and about the ankle erythema, with distention, and small bullae (phlyctaenae); acute fever; he became furiously deranged; alvine discharges bilious, unmixed, and rather frequent. He died on the second day from the commencement.

CASE X. The Clazomenian who was lodged by the Well of Phrynichides was seized with fever. He had pain in the head, neck, and loins from the beginning, and immediately afterwards deafness; no sleep, acute fever, hypochondria elevated with a swelling, but not much distention; tongue dry. On the fourth, towards night, he became delirious. On the fifth, in an uneasy state. On the sixth, all the symptoms exacerbated. About the eleventh a slight remission; from the commencement to the fourteenth day the alvine discharges thin, copious, and of the color of water, but were well supported; the bowels then became constipated. Urine throughout thin, and well colored, and had many substances scattered through it, but no sediment. About the sixteenth, urine somewhat thicker, which had a slight sediment; somewhat better, and more collected. On the seventeenth, urine again thin; swellings about both his ears, with pain; no sleep, some incoherence; legs painfully affected. On the twentieth, free of fever, had a crisis, no sweat, perfectly collected. About the twenty-seventh, violent pain of the right hip; it speedily went off. The swellings about the ears subsided, and did not suppurate, but were painful. About the thirty-first, a diarrhea attended with a copious discharge of watery matter, and symptoms of dysentery; passed thick urine; swellings about the ears gone. About the fortieth day, had pain in the right eye, sight dull. It went away.

CASE XI. The wife of Dromeades having been delivered of a female child, and all other matters going on properly, on the second day after was seized with rigor and acute fever. Began to have pain about the hypochondrium on the first day; had nausea and incoherence, and for some hours afterwards had no sleep; respiration rare, large, and suddenly interrupted. On the day following that on which she had the rigor, alvine discharges proper; urine thick, white, muddy, like urine which has been shaken after standing for some time, until the sediment had fallen to the bottom; it had no sediment; she did not sleep during the night. On the third day, about noon, had a rigor, acute fever; urine the same; pain of the hypochondria, nausea, an uncomfortable night, no sleep; a coldish sweat all over, but heat quickly restored. On the fourth, slight alleviation of the symptoms about the hypochondria; heaviness of the head, with pain; somewhat comatose; slight epistaxis, tongue dry, thirst, urine thin and oily; slept a little, upon awaking was somewhat comatose; slight coldness, slept during the night, was delirious. On the morning of the sixth had a rigor, but soon recovered her heat, sweated all over; extremities cold, was delirious, respiration rare and large. Shortly afterwards spasms from the head began, and she immediately expired.

CASE XII. A man, in a heated state, took supper, and drank more than enough; he vomited the whole during the night; acute fever, pain of the right hypochondrium, a softish inflammation from the inner part; passed an uncomfortable night; urine at the commencement thick, red, but when allowed to stand, had no sediment, tongue dry, and not very thirsty. On the fourth, acute fever, pains all over. On the fifth, urine smooth, oily, and copious; acute fever. On the sixth, in the evening, very incoherent, no sleep during the night. On the seventh, all the symptoms exacerbated; urine of the same characters; much talking, and he could not contain himself; the bowels being stimulated, passed a watery discharge with lumbrici: night equally painful. In the morning had a rigor; acute fever, hot sweat, appeared to be free of fever; did not sleep long; after the sleep a chill, ptyalism; in the evening, great incoherence; after a little, vomited a small quantity of dark bilious matters. On the ninth, coldness, much delirium, did not sleep. On the tenth, pains in the limbs, all the symptoms exacerbated; he was delirious. On the eleventh, he died.

CASE XIII. A woman, who lodged on the Quay, being three months gone with child, was seized with fever, and immediately began to have pains in the loins. On the third day, pain of the head and neck, extending to the clavicle, and right hand; she immediately lost the power of speech; was paralyzed in the right hand, with spasms, after the manner of paraplegia; was quite incoherent; passed an uncomfortable night; did not sleep; disorder of the bowels, attended with bilious, On the fourth, recovered the use of her tongue; spasms of the same parts, and general pains remained; swelling in the hypochondrium, accompanied with pain; did not sleep, was quite incoherent; bowels disordered, urine thin, and not of a good color. On the fifth, acute fever; pain of the hypochondrium, quite incoherent; alvine evacuations bilious; towards night had a sweat, and was freed from the fever. On the sixth, recovered her reason; was every way relieved; the pain remained about the left clavicle; was thirsty, urine thin, had no sleep. On the seventh trembling, slight coma, some incoherence, pains about the clavicle and left arm remained; in all other respects was alleviated; quite coherent. For three days remained free from fever. On the eleventh, had a relapse, with rigor and fever. About the fourteenth day, vomited pretty abundantly bilious and yellow matters, had a sweat, the fever went off, by coming to a crisis.

CASE XIV. Melidia, who lodged near the Temple of Juno, began to feel a violent pain of the head, neck, and chest. She was straightway seized with acute fever; a slight appearance of the menses; continued pains of all these parts. On the sixth, was affected with coma, nausea, and rigor; redness about the cheeks; slight delirium. On the seventh, had a sweat; the fever intermitted, the pains remained. A relapse; little sleep; urine throughout of a good color, but thin; the alvine evacuations were thin, bilious, acrid, very scanty, black, and fetid; a white, smooth sediment in the urine; had a sweat, and experienced a perfect crisis on the eleventh day.

BOOK II.

Sect. I

CASE I. Pythion, who lived by the Temple of the Earth, on the first day, trembling commencing from his hands; acute fever, delirium. On the second, all the symptoms were exacerbated. On the third, the same. On the fourth alvine discharges scanty, unmixed, and bilious. On the fifth, all the symptoms were exacerbated, the tremors remained; little sleep, the bowels constipated. On the sixth sputa mixed, reddish. On the seventh, mouth drawn aside. On the eighth, all the symptoms were exacerbated; the tremblings were again constant; urine, from the beginning to the eighth day, thin, and devoid of color; substances floating in it, cloudy. On the tenth he sweated; sputa somewhat digested, had a crisis; urine thinnish about the crisis; but after the crisis, on the fortieth day, an abscess about the anus, which passed off by a strangury.

Explanation of the characters. It is probably that the great discharge of urine brought about the resolution of the disease, and the cure of the patient on the fortieth day.

CASE II. Hermocrates, who lived by the New Wall, was seized with fever. He began to have pain in the head and loins; an empty distention of the hypochondrium; the tongue at first was parched; deafness at the commencement; there was no sleep; not very thirsty; urine thick and red, when allowed to stand it did not subside; alvine discharge very dry, and not scanty. On the fifth, urine thin, had substances floating in it which did not fall to the bottom; at night he was delirious. On the sixth, had jaundice; all the symptoms were exacerbated; had no recollection. On the seventh, in an uncomfortable state; urine thin, as formerly;

on the following days the same. About the eleventh day, all the symptoms appeared to be lightened. Coma set in; urine thicker, reddish, thin substances below, had no sediment; by degrees he became collected. On the fourteenth, fever gone; had no sweat; slept, quite collected; urine of the same characters. About the seventeenth, had a relapse, became hot. On the following days, acute fever, urine thin, was delirious. Again, on the twentieth, had a crisis; free of fever; had no sweat; no appetite through the whole time; was perfectly collected; could not speak, tongue dry, without thirst; deep sleep. About the twenty-fourth day he became heated; bowels loose, with a thin, watery discharge; on the following days acute fever, tongue parched. On the twenty-seventh he died. In this patient deafness continued throughout; the urine either thick and red, without sediment, or thin, devoid of color, and, having substances floating in it: he could taste nothing.

Explanation of the characters. It is probably that it was the suppression of the discharges from the bowels which occasioned death on the twenty-seventh day.

CASE III. The man who was lodged in the Garden of Dealces: had heaviness of the head and pain in the right temple for a considerable time, from some accidental cause, was seized with fever, and took to bed. On the second, there was a trickling of pure blood from the left nostril, but the alvine discharges were proper, urine thin, mixed, having small substances floating in it, like coarse barley meal, or semen. On the third, acute fever; stools black, thin, frothy, a livid sediment in the dejections; slight coma; uneasiness at the times he had to get up; sediment in the urine livid, and somewhat viscid. On the fourth, slight vomiting of bilious, yellow matters, and, after a short interval, of the color of verdigris; a few drops of pure blood ran from the left nostril; stools the same; urine the same; sweated about the head and clavicles; spleen enlarged, pain of the thigh on the same side; loose swelling of the right hypochondrium; at night had no sleep, slight delirium. On the sixth, stools black, fatty, viscid, fetid; slept, more collected. On the seventh, tongue dry, thirsty, did not sleep; was somewhat delirious; urine thin, not of a good color. On the eighth, stools black, scanty, and compact; slept, became collected; not very thirsty. On the ninth had a rigor, acute fever, sweated, a chill, was delirious, strabismus of the right eye, tongue dry, thirsty, without sleep. On the tenth, much the same. On the eleventh, became quite collected; free from fever, slept, urine thin about the crisis. The two following days without fever; it returned on the fourteenth, then immediately insomnolency and complete delirium. On the fifteenth, urine muddy, like that which has been shaken after the sediment has fallen to the bottom; acute fever, quite delirious, did not sleep; knees and legs painful; after a suppository, had alvine dejections of a black color. On the sixteenth, urine thin, had a cloudy eneorema, was delirious. On the seventeenth, in the morning, extremities cold, was covered up with the bedclothes, acute fever, general sweat, felt relieved, more collected; not free of fever, thirsty, vomited yellow bile, in small quantities; formed faeces passed from the bowels, but soon afterwards black, scanty, and thin; urine thin, not well colored. On the eighteenth, not collected, comatose. On the nineteenth, in the same state. On the twentieth, slept; quite collected, sweated, free from fever, not thirsty, but the urine thin. On the twenty-first, slight delirium; somewhat thirsty, pain of the hypochondrium, and throbbing about the navel throughout. On sediment in the urine, quite collected. Twenty-seventh, pain of the right hip joint; urine thin and bad, a sediment; all the other symptoms milder. About the twenty-ninth, pain of the right eye; urine thin. Fortieth, dejections pituitous, white, rather frequent; sweated abundantly all over; had a complete crisis.

Explanation of the characters. It is probable that, by means of the stools, the urine, and the sweat, this patient was cured in forty days.

Sect. II

CASE I. In Thasus, Philistes had headache of long continuance, and sometimes was confined to bed, with a tendency to deep sleep; having been seized with continual fevers from drinking, the pain was exacerbated; during the night he, at first, became hot. On the first day, he vomited some bilious matters, at first yellow, but afterwards of a verdigris-green color, and in greater quantity; formed faeces passed from the bowels; passed the night uncomfortably. On the second, deafness, acute fever; retraction of the right hypochondrium; urine thin, transparent, had some small substances like semen floating in it; delirium ferox about mid-day. On the third, in an uncomfortable state. On the fourth, convulsions; all the symptoms exacerbated. On the fifth, early in the morning, died.

Explanation of the characters. It is probable that the death of the patient on the fifth day is to be attributed to a phrenitis, with unfavorable evacuations.

CASE II. Charion, who was lodged at the house of Demaenetus, contracted a fever from drinking. Immediately he had a painful heaviness of the head; did not sleep; bowels disordered, with thin and somewhat bilious discharges. On the third day, acute fever; trembling of the head, but especially of the lower lip; after a little time a rigor, convulsions; he was quite delirious; passed the night uncomfortably. On the fourth, quiet, slept little, talked incoherently. On the fifth, in pain; all the symptoms exacerbated; delirium; passed the night uncomfortably; did not sleep. On the sixth, in the same state. On the seventh had a rigor, acute fever, sweated all over his body; had a crisis. Throughout the alvine discharges were bilious, scanty, and unmixed; urine thin, well colored, having cloudy substances floating in it. About the eighth day, passed urine of a better color, having a white scanty sediment; was collected, free from fever for a season. On the ninth it relapsed. About the fourteenth, acute fever. On the sixteenth, vomited pretty frequently yellow, bilious matters. On the seventeenth had a rigor, acute fever, sweated, free of fever; had a crisis; urine, after the relapse and the crisis, well colored, having a sediment; neither was he delirious in the relapse. On the eighteenth, became a little heated; some thirst, urine thin, with cloudy substances floating in it; slight wandering in his mind. About the nineteenth, free of fever, had a pain in his neck; a sediment in the urine. Had a complete crisis on the twentieth.

Explanation of the characters. It is probable that the patient was cured in twenty days, by the abundance of bilious stools and urine.

CASE III. The daughter of Euryanax, a maid, was taken ill of fever. She was free of thirst throughout, but had no relish for food. Alvine discharges small, urine thin, scanty, not well colored. In the beginning of the fever, had a pain about the nates. On the sixth day, was free of fever, did not sweat, had a crisis; the complaint about the nates came to a small suppuration, and burst at the crisis. After the crisis, on the seventh day, had a rigor, became slightly heated, sweated. On the eighth day after the rigor, had an inconsiderable rigor; the extremities cold ever after. About the tenth day, after a sweat which came on, she became delirious, and again immediately afterwards was collected; these symptoms were said to have been brought on by eating grapes. After an intermission of the twelfth day, she again talked much incoherently; her bowels disordered with bilious, scanty, unmixed, thin, acrid discharges; she required to get frequently up. She died on the seventh day after the return of the delirium. At the commencement of the disease she had pain in the throat, and it red throughout, uvula retracted, defluxions abundant, thin, acrid; coughed, but had no concocted sputa; during the whole time loathed all kinds of food, nor had the least desire of anything; had no thirst, nor drank anything worth mentioning; was silent, and never spoke a word; despondency; had no hopes of herself. She had a congenital tendency to phthisis.

CASE IV. The woman affected with quinsy, who lodged in the house of Aristion: her complaint began in the tongue; speech inarticulate; tongue red and parched. On the first day, felt chilly, and afterwards became heated. On the third day, a rigor, acute fever; a reddish and hard swelling on both sides of the neck and chest, extremities cold and livid; and livid; respiration elevated; the drink returned by the nose; she could not swallow; alvine and urinary discharges suppressed. On the fourth, all of the symptoms were exacerbated. On the fifth she died of the quinsy.

Explanation of the characters. It is probable that the cause of death on the sixth day was the suppression of the discharges.

CASE V. The young man who was lodged by the Liars' Market was seized with fever from fatigue, labor, and running out of season. On the first day, the bowels disordered, with bilious, thin, and copious dejections; urine thin and blackish; had no sleep; was thirsty. On the second all the symptoms were exacerbated; dejections more copious and unseasonable; he had no sleep; disorder of the intellect; slight sweat. On the third day, restless, thirst, nausea, much tossing about, bewilderment, delirium; extremities livid and cold; softish distention of the hypochondrium on both sides. On the fourth, did not sleep; still worse. On the seventh he died. He was about twenty years of age.

Explanation of the characters. It is probable that the cause of his death on the seventh day was the unseasonable practices mentioned above. An acute affection.

CASE VI. The woman who lodged at the house of Tisamenas had a troublesome attack of iliac passion, much vomiting; could not keep her drink; pains about the hypochondria, and pains also in the lower part of the belly; constant tormina; not thirsty; became hot; extremities cold throughout, with nausea and insomnolency; urine scanty and thin; dejections undigested, thin, scanty. Nothing could do her any good. She died.

CASE VII. A woman of Pantimides, from a miscarriage, was taken ill of fever. On the first day, tongue dry, thirst, nausea, insomnolency, belly disordered, with thin, copious, undigested dejections. On the second day, had a rigor, acute fever; alvine discharges copious; had no sleep. On the third, pains greater. On the fourth, delirious. On the seventh she died. Belly throughout loose, with copious, thin, undigested evacuations; urine scanty, thin. An ardent fever.

CASE VIII. Another woman, after a miscarriage about the fifth month, the wife of Ocetes, was seized with fever. At first had sometimes coma and sometimes insomnolency; pain of the loins; heaviness of the head. On the second, the bowels were disordered, with scanty, thin, and at first unmixed dejections. On the third, more copious, and worse; at night did not sleep. On the fourth was delirious; frights, despondency; strabismus of the right eye; a faint cold sweat about the head; extremities cold. On the fifth day, all the symptoms were exacerbated; talked much incoherently, and again immediately became collected; had no thirst; labored under insomnolency; alvine dejections copious, and unseasonable throughout; urine scanty, thin, darkish; extremities cold, somewhat livid. On the sixth day, in the same state. On the seventh she died. Phrenitis.

CASE IX. A woman who lodged near the Liars' Market, having then brought forth a son in a first and difficult labor, was seized with fever. Immediately on the commencement had thirst, nausea, and cardialgia; tongue dry; bowels disordered, with thin and scanty dejections; had no sleep. On the second, had slight rigor, acute fever; a faint cold sweat about the head. On the third, painfully affected; evacuations from the bowels undigested, thin, and copious. On the fourth, had a rigor; all the symptoms exacerbated; insomnolency. On the fifth, in a painful state. On the sixth, in the same state; discharges from the bowels liquid and copious. On the seventh, had a rigor, fever acute; much thirst; much tossing about; towards evening a cold sweat over all; extremities cold, could no longer be kept warm; and again at night had a rigor; extremities could not be warmed; she did not sleep; was slightly delirious, and again speedily collected. On the eighth, about mid-day, she became warm, was thirsty, comatose, had nausea; vomited small quantities of yellowish bile; restless at night, did not sleep; passed frequently large quantities of urine without consciousness. On the ninth, all the symptoms gave way; comatose, towards evening slight rigors; small vomitings of bile. On the tenth, rigor; exacerbation of the fever, did not sleep at all; in the morning passed much urine having a sediment; extremities recovered their heat. On the eleventh, vomited bile of a verdigris-green color; not long after had a rigor, and again the extremities cold; towards evening a rigor, a cold sweat, much vomiting; passed a painful night. On the twelfth, had copious black and fetid vomitings; much hiccup, painful thirst. On the thirteenth, vomitings black, fetid, and copious; rigor about mid-day, loss of speech. On the fourteenth, some blood ran from her nose, she died. In this case the bowels were loose throughout; with rigors: her age about seventeen. An ardent fever.

Sect. III

1. The year was southerly, rainy; no winds throughout. Droughts having prevailed during the previous seasons of the year, the south winds towards the rising of Arcturus were attended with much rain. Autumn gloomy and cloudy, with copious rains. Winter southerly, damp, and soft. But long after the solstice, and near the equinox, much wintery weather out of season; and when now close to the equinox, northerly, and winterly weather for no long time. The spring again southerly, calm, much rain until the dog-days. Summer fine and hot; great suffocating heats. The Etesian winds blew small and irregular; again, about the season of Arcturus, much rains with north winds.

2. The year being southerly, damp, and soft towards winter, all were healthy, except those affected with phthisis, of whom we shall write afterwards.

3. Early in spring, along with the prevailing cold, there were many cases of erysipelas, some from a manifest cause, and some not. They were of a malignant nature, and proved fatal to many; many had sore-throat and loss of speech. There were many cases of ardent fever, phrensy, aphthous affections of the mouth, tumors on the genital organs; of ophthalmia, anthrax, disorder of the bowels, anorexia, with thirst and without it; of disordered urine, large in quantity, and bad in quality; of persons affected with coma for a long time, and then falling into a state of insomnolency. There were many cases of failure of crisis, and many of unfavorable crisis; many of dropsy and of phthisis. Such were the diseases then epidemic. There were patients affected with every one of the species which have been mentioned, and many died. The symptoms in each of these cases were as follows:

4. In many cases erysipelas, from some obvious cause, such as an accident, and sometimes from even a very small wound, broke out all over the body, especially, in persons about sixty years of age, about the head, if such an accident was neglected in the slightest degree; and this happened in some who were under treatment; great inflammation took place, and the erysipelas quickly spread all over. in the most of them abscessed ended in suppurations, and there were great fallings off (sloughing) of the flesh, tendons, and bones; and the defluxion which seated in the part was not like pus, but a sort of putrefaction, and the running was large and of various characters. Those cases in which any of these things happened about the head were accompanied with falling off of the hairs of the head and chin, the bones were laid bare and separated, and there were excessive runnings; and these symptoms happened in fevers and without fevers. But these things were more formidable in appearance than dangerous; for when the concoction in these cases turned to a these cases turned to a suppuration, most of them recovered; but when the inflammation and erysipelas disappeared, and when no abscess was formed, a great number of these died. In like manner, the same things happened to whatever part of the body the disease wandered, for in many cases both forearm and arm dropped off; and in those cases in which it fell upon the sides, the parts there, either before or behind, got into a bad state; and in some cases the whole femur and bones of the leg and whole foot were laid bare. But of all such cases, the most formidable were those which took place about the pubes and genital organs. Such was the nature of these cases when attended with sores, and proceeding from an external cause; but the same things occurred in fevers, before fevers, and after fevers. fevers. But those cases in which an abscess was formed, and turned to a suppuration, or a seasonable diarrhea or discharge of good urine took place, were relieved thereby: but those cases in which none of these symptoms occurred, but they disappeared without a crisis, proved fatal. The greater number of these erysipelatous cases took place in the spring, but were prolonged through the summer and during autumn.

5. In certain cases there was much disorder, and tumors about the fauces, and inflammations of the tongue, and abscesses about the teeth. And many were attacked with impairment or loss of speech; at first, those in the commencement of phthisis, but also persons in ardent fever and in phrenitis.

6. The cases of ardent fever and phrenitis occurred early in spring after the cold set in, and great numbers were taken ill at that time, and these cases were attended with acute and fatal symptoms. The constitution of the ardent fevers which then occurred was as follows: at the commencement they were affected with coma, nausea, and rigors; fever acute, not much thirst, nor delirium, slight epistaxis, the paroxysms for the most part on even days; and, about the time of the paroxysms, forgetfulness, loss of strength and of speech, the extremities, that is to say, the hands and feet, at all times, but more especially about the time of the paroxysms, were colder than natural; they slowly and imperfectly became warmed, and again recovered their recollection and speech. They were constantly affected either with coma, in which they got which they got no sleep, or with insomnolency, attended with pains; most had disorders of the bowels, attended with undigested, thin, and copious evacuations; urine copious, thin, having nothing critical nor favorable about it; neither was there any other critical appearance in persons affected thus; for

neither was there any proper hemorrhage, nor any other of the accustomed evacuations, to prove a crisis. They died, as it happened, in an irregular manner, mostly about the crisis, but in some instances after having lost their speech for a long time, and having had copious sweats. These were the symptoms which marked the fatal cases of ardent fever; similar symptoms occurred in the phrenitic cases; but these were particularly free from thirst, and none of these had wild delirium as in other cases, but they died oppressed by a bad tendency to sleep, and stupor.

7. But there were also other fevers, as will be described. Many had their mouths affected with aphthous ulcerations. There were also many defluxions about the genital parts, and ulcerations, boils (phymata), externally and internally, about the groins. Watery ophthalmies of a chronic character, with pains; fungous excrescences of the eyelids, externally and internally, called fig, which destroyed the sight of many persons. There were fungous growths, in many other instances, on ulcers, especially on those seated on the genital organs. There were many attacks of carbuncle (anthrax) through the summer, and other affections, which are called "the putrefaction" (seps); also large ecthymata, and large tetters (herpetes) in many instances.

8. And many and serious complaints attacked many persons in the region of the belly. In the first place, tenesmus, accompanied with pain, attacked many, but more especially children, and all who had not attained to puberty; and the most of these died. There were many cases of lientery and of dysentery; but these were not attended with much pain. The evacuations were bilious, and fatty, and thin, and watery; in many instances the disease terminated in this way, with and without fever; there were painful tormina and volvuli of a malignant kind; copious evacuations of the contents of the guts, and yet much remained behind; and

the passages did not carry off the pains, but yielded with difficulty to the means administered; for in most cases purgings were hurtful to those affected in this manner; many died speedily, but in many others they held out longer. In a word, all died, both those who had acute attacks and those who had chronic, most especially from affections of the belly, for it was the belly which carried them all off.

9. All persons had an aversion to food in all the afore-mentioned complaints to a degree such as I never met with before, and persons in these complaints most especially, and those recovering from them, and in all other diseases of a mortal nature. Some were troubled with thirst, and some not; and both in febrile complaints and in others no one drank unseasonably or disobeyed injunctions.

10. The urine in many cases was not in proportion to the drink administered, but greatly in excess; and the badness of the urine voided was great, for it had not the proper thickness, nor concoction, nor purged properly; for in many cases purgings by the bladder indicate favorably, but in the greatest number they indicated a melting of the body, disorder of the bowels, pains, and a want of crisis.

11. Persons laboring under phrenitis and causus were particularly disposed to coma; but also in all other great diseases which occurred along with fever. In the main, most cases were attended either by heavy coma, or by short and light sleep.

12. And many other forms of fevers were then epidemic, of tertian, of quartan, of nocturnal, of continual, of chronic, of erratic, of fevers attended with nausea, and of irregular fevers. All these were attended with much disorder, for the bowels in most cases were disordered, accompanied with rigors, sweats not of a critical character, and with the state of the urine as described. In most instances the disease was protracted, for neither did the deposits which took place prove critical as in other cases; for in all complaints and in all cases there was difficulty of crisis, want of crisis, and protraction of the disease, but most especially in these. A few had the crisis about the eightieth day, but in most instances it (the disease?) left them irregularly. A few of them died of dropsy without being confined to bed. And in many other diseases people were troubled with swelling, but more especially in phthisical cases.

13. The greatest and most dangerous disease, and the one that proved fatal to the greatest number, was consumption. With many persons it commenced during the winter, and of these some were confined to bed, and others bore up on foot; the most of those died early in spring who were confined to bed; of the others, the cough left not a single person, but it became milder through the summer; during the autumn, all these were confined to bed, and many of them died, but in the greater number of cases the disease was long protracted. Most of these were suddenly attacked with these diseases, having frequent rigors, often continual and acute fevers; unseasonable, copious, and cold sweats throughout; great coldness, from which they had great difficulty in being restored to heat; the bowels variously constipated, and again immediately in a loose state, but towards the termination in all cases with violent looseness of the bowels; a determination downwards of all matters collected about the lungs; urine excessive, and not good; troublesome melting. The coughs throughout were frequent, and copious, digested, and liquid, but not brought up with much pain; and even when they had some slight pain, in all cases the purging of the matters about the lungs went on mildly. The fauces were not very irritable, nor were they troubled with any saltish humors; but there were viscid, white, liquid, frothy, and copious defluxions from the head. But by far the greatest mischief attending these and the other complaints, was the aversion to food, as has been described. For neither been described. For neither had they any relish for drink along with their food, but continued without thirst. There was heaviness of the body, disposition to coma, in most cases swelling, which ended in dropsy; they had rigors, and were delirious towards death.

14. The form of body peculiarly subject to phthisical complaints was the smooth, the whitish, that resembling the lentil; the reddish, the blue-eyed, the leucophlegmatic, and that with the scapulae having the appearance of wings: and women in like manner, with regard to the melancholic and subsanguineous, phrenitic and dysenteric affections principally attacked them. Tenesmus troubled young persons of a phlegmatic temperament. Chronic diarrhoea, acrid and viscid discharges from the bowels, attacked those who were troubled with bitter bile.

15. To all those which have been described, the season of spring was most inimical, and proved fatal to the greatest numbers: the summer was the most favorable to them, and the fewest died then; in autumn, and under the Pleiades, again there died great numbers. It appears to me, according to the reason of things, that the coming on of summer should have done good in these cases; for winter coming on cures the diseases of summer, and summer coming on removes the diseases of winter. And yet the summer in question was not of itself well constituted, for it became suddenly hot, southerly, and calm; but, not withstanding, it proved beneficial by producing a change on the other constitution.

16. I look upon it as being a great part of the art to be able to judge properly of that which has been written. For he that knows and makes a proper use of these things, would appear to me not likely to commit any great mistake in the art. He ought to learn accurately the constitution of every one of the seasons, and of the diseases; whatever that is common in each constitution and disease is good, and whatever is bad; whatever disease will be protracted and end in death, and whatever will be protracted and end in recovery; which disease of an acute nature will end in death, and which in recovery. From these it is easy to know the order of the critical days, and prognosticate from them accordingly. And to a person who is skilled in these things, it is easy to know to whom, when, and how aliment ought to be administered.

Sixteen Cases of Disease

CASE I. In Thasus, the Parian who lodged above the Temple of Diana was seized with an acute fever, at first of a continual and ardent type; thirsty, inclined to be comatose at first, and afterwards troubled with insomnolency; bowels disordered at the beginning, urine thin. On the sixth day, passed oily urine, was delirious. On the seventh, all the symptoms were exacerbated; had no sleep, but the urine of the same characters, and the understanding disordered; alvine dejections bilious and fatty. On the eighth, a slight epistaxis; small vomiting of verdigris-green matters; slept a little. On the ninth, in the same state. On the tenth, all the symptoms gave way. On the eleventh, he sweated, but not over the whole body; he became cold, but immediately recovered his heat again. On the fourteenth, acute fever; discharges bilious, thin, and copious; substances floating in the urine; he became incoherent. On the seventeenth, in a painful state, for he had no sleep, and the fever was more intense. On the twentieth, sweated all over; apyrexia, dejections bilious; aversion to food, comatose. On the twenty-fourth, had a relapse. On the thirty-fourth, apyrexia; bowels not confined; and he again recovered his heat. Fortieth, apyrexia, bowels confined for no long time, aversion to food; had again slight symptoms of fever, and throughout in an irregular form; apyrexia at times, and at others not; for if the fever intermitted, and was alleviated for a little, it immediately relapsed again; he used much and improper food; sleep bad; about the time of the relapse he was delirious; passed thick urine at that time, but troubled, and of bad characters; bowels at first confined, and again loose; slight fevers of a continual type; discharges copious and thin. On the hundred and twentieth day he died. In this patient the bowels were constantly from the first either loose, with bilious, liquid, and copious dejections, or constipated with hot and undigested faeces; the urine throughout bad; for the most part coma, or insomnolency with pain; continued aversion to food. Ardent fever.

Explanation of the characters. It is probable that the weakness produced by the fever, the phrenitis, and affection of the hypochondrium caused death on the hundred and twentieth day.

CASE II. In Thasus, the woman who lodged near the Cold Water, on the third day after delivery of a daughter, the lochial discharge not taking place, was seized with acute fever, accompanied with rigors. But a considerable time before delivery she was feverish, confined to bed, and loathed her food. After the rigor which took place, continual and acute fevers, with rigors. On the eighth and following days, was very incoherent, and immediately afterwards became collected; bowels disordered, with copious, thin, watery, and bilious stools; no thirst. On the eleventh was collected, but disposed to coma; urine copious, thin, and black; no sleep. On the twentieth, slight chills, and immediately afterwards was warm; slight incoherence; no sleep; with regard to the bowels, in the same condition; urine watery, and copious. On the twenty-seventh, free from fever; bowels constipated; not long afterwards violent pain of the right hip-joint for a considerable time; fevers afterwards supervened; urine watery. On the fortieth, complaints about the hip-joint better; continued coughs, with copious, watery sputa; bowels constipated; aversion to food; urine the same; fever not leaving her entirely, but having paroxysms in an irregular form, sometimes present, sometimes not. On the sixtieth, the coughs left her without a crisis, for no concoction of the sputa took place, nor any of the usual abscesses; jaw on the right side convulsively retracted; comatose, was again incoherent, and immediately became collected; utter aversion to food; the jaw became relaxed; alvine discharges small, and bilious; fever more acute, affected with rigors; on the following days lost her speech, and again became collected, and talked. On the eightieth she died. In this case the urine throughout was black, thin, and watery; coma supervened; there was aversion to food, aversion to food, despondency, and insomnolency; irritability, restlessness; she was of a melancholic turn of mind.

Explanation of the characters. It is probable that the suppression of the lochial discharge caused death on the day.

CASE III. In Thasus, Pythion, who was lodged above the Temple of Hercules, from labor, fatigue, and neglected diet, was seized with strong rigor and acute fever; tongue dry, thirsty, and bilious; had no sleep; urine darkish, eneorema floating on the top of the urine, did not subside. On the second day, about noon, coldness of the extremities, especially about the hands and head; loss of speech and of articulation; breathing short for a considerable time; recovered his heat; thirst; passed the night quietly; slight sweats about the head. On the third, passed the day in a composed state; in the evening, about sunset, slight chills; nausea, agitation; passed the night in a painful state; had no sleep; small stools of compact faeces passed from the bowels. On the fourth, in the morning, composed; about noon all the symptoms became exacerbated; coldness, loss of speech, and of articulation; became worse; recovered his heat after a time; passed black urine, having substances floating in it; the night quiet; slept. On the fifth, seemed to be lightened, but a painful weight about the belly; thirsty, passed the night in a painful state. On the sixth, in the morning, in a quiet state; in the evening the pains greater; had a paroxysm; in the evening the bowels properly opened by a small clyster; slept at night. On the seventh, during the day, in a state of nausea, somewhat disturbed; passed urine of the appearance of oil; at night, much agitation, was incoherent, did not sleep. On the eighth, in the morning, slept a little; but immediately coldness, loss of speech, respiration small and weak; but in the evening recovered his heat again; was delirious, but towards day was somewhat lightened; stools small, bilious, and unmixed. On the ninth, affected with coma, and with nausea when roused; not very thirsty; about sunset he became restless and incoherent; passed a bad night. On the tenth, in the morning, had become speechless; great coldness; acute fever; much perspiration; he died. His sufferings were on the even days.

Explanation of the characters. It is probable that the excessive sweats caused death on the tenth day.

CASE IV. The patient affected with phrenitis, having taken to bed on the first day, vomited largely of verdigris-green and thin matters; fever, accompanied with rigors, copious and continued sweats all over; heaviness of the head and neck, with pain; urine thin, substances floating in the urine small, scattered, did not subside; had copious dejections from the bowels; very delirious; no sleep. On the second, in the morning, loss of speech;

acute fever; he sweated, fever did not leave him; palpitations over the whole body, at night, convulsions. On the third, all the symptoms exacerbated; he died.

Explanation of the characters. It is probable that the sweats and convulsions caused death.

CASE V. In Larissa, a man, who was bald, suddenly was seized with pain in the right thigh; none of the things which were administered did him any good. On the first day, fever acute, of the ardent type, not agitated, but the pains persisted. On the second, the pains in the thigh abated, but the fever increased; somewhat tossed about; did not sleep; extremities cold; passed a large quantity of urine, not of a good character. On the third, the pain of the thigh ceased; derangement of the intellect, confusion, and much tossing about. On the fourth, about noon, he died. An acute disease.

CASE VI. In Abdera, Pericles was seized with a fever of the acute, continual type, with pain; much thirst, nausea, could not retain his drink; somewhat swelled about the spleen, with heaviness of the head. On the first day, had hemorrhage from the left nostril, but still the fever became more violent; passed much muddy, white urine, which when allowed to stand did not subside. On the second day, all the symptoms were exacerbated, yet the urine was thick, and more inclined to have a sediment; the nausea less; he slept. On the third, fever was milder; abundance of urine, which was concocted, and had a copious sediment; passed a quiet night. On the fourth, had a copious and warm sweat all over about noon; was free of fever, had a crisis, no relapse. An acute affection.

CASE VII. In Abdera, the young woman who was lodged in the Sacred Walk was seized with an ardent fever. She was thirsty, and could not sleep; had menstruation for the first time. On the sixth, much nausea, flushing, was chilly, and tossed about. On the seventh, in the same state; urine thin, but of a good color; no disturbance about the bowels. On the eighth, deafness, acute fever, insomnolency, nausea, rigors, became collected; urine the same. On the ninth, in the same state, and also on the following days; thus the deafness persisted. On the fourteenth, disorder of the intellect; the fever abated. On the seventeenth, a copious hemorrhage from the nose; the deafness slightly better; and on the following days, nausea, deafness, and incoherence. On the twentieth, pain of the feet; deafness and delirium left her; a small hemorrhage from the nose; sweat, apyrexia. On the twenty-fourth, the fever returned, deafness again; pain of the feet remained; incoherence. On the twenty-seventh, had a copious sweat, apyrexia; the deafness left her; the pain of her feet partly remained; in other respects had a complete crisis.

Explanation of the characters. It is probable that the restoration of health on the twentieth day was the result of the evacuation of urine.

CASE VIII. In Abdera, Anaxion, who was lodged near the with Thracian Gates, was seized with an acute fever; pain of the right dry cough, without expectoration during the first days, thirst, insomnolency; urine well colored, copious, and thin. On the sixth, delirious; no relief from the warm applications. On the seventh, in a painful state, for the fever while the pains did not abate, and the cough was troublesome, and attended with dyspnoea. On the eighth, I opened a vein at the elbow, and much blood, of a proper character, flowed; the pains were abated, but the dry coughs continued. On the eleventh, the fever diminished; slight sweats about the head; coughs, with more liquid sputa; he was relieved. On the twentieth, sweat, apyrexia; but after the crisis he was thirsty, and the expectorations were not good. On the twenty-seventh the fever relapsed; he coughed, and brought up much concocted sputa: sediment in the urine copious and white; he became free of thirst, and the respiration was good. On the thirty-fourth, sweated all over, apyrexia general crisis.

Explanation of the characters. It is probable that the evacuation of the sputa brought about the recovery on the thirty-fourth day.

CASE IX. In Abdera, Heropythus, while still on foot, had pain in the head, and not long afterwards he took to bed; he lived near the High Street. Was seized with acute fever of the ardent type; vomitings at first of much bilious matter; thirst; great restlessness; urine thin, black, substances sometimes floating high in it, and sometimes not; passed the night in a painful state; paroxysms of the fever diversified, and for the most part irregular. About the fourteenth day, deafness; the fever increased; urine the same. On the twentieth and following days, much delirium. On the thirtieth, copious hemorrhage from the nose, and became more collected; deafness continued, but less; the fever diminished; on the following days, frequent hemorrhages, at short intervals. About the sixtieth, the hemorrhages ceased, but violent pain of the hip-joint, and increase of fever. Not long afterwards, pains of all the inferior rule, that either the fever and deafness increased, or, pains of the inferior parts were increased. About the eightieth day, all the complaints gave way, without leaving any behind; for the urine was of a good color, and had a copious sediment, while the delirium became less. About the hundredth day, disorder of the bowels, with copious and bilious evacuations, and these continued for a considerable time, and again assumed the dysenteric form with pain; but relief of all the other complaints. On the whole, the fevers went off, and the deafness ceased. On the hundred and twentieth day, had a complete crisis. Ardent fever.

Explanation of the characters. It is probable that the bilious discharge brought about the recovery on the hundred and twentieth day.

CASE X. In Abdera, Nicodemus was seized with fever from venery and drinking. At the commencement he was troubled with nausea and cardialgia; thirsty, tongue was parched; urine thin and dark. On the second day, the fever exacerbated; he was troubled with rigors and nausea; had no sleep; vomited yellow bile; urine the same; passed a quiet night, and slept. On the third, a general remission; amelioration; but about sunset felt again somewhat uncomfortable; passed an uneasy night. On the fourth, rigor, much fever, general pains; urine thin, with substances floating in it; again a quiet night. On the fifth, all the symptoms remained, but there was an amelioration. On the sixth, some general pains; substances floating in the urine; very incoherent. On the seventh, better. On the eighth, all the other symptoms abated. On the tenth, and following days, there were pains, but all less; in this case throughout, the paroxysms and pains were greater on the even days. On the twentieth, the urine white and thick, but when allowed to stand had no sediment; much sweat; seemed to be free from fever; but again in the evening he became hot, with the same pains, rigor, thirst, slightly incoherent. On the twenty-fourth, urine copious, white, with an abundant sediment; a copious and warm sweat all over; apyrexia; the fever came to its crisis.

Explanation of the characters. It is probable that the cure was owing to the bilious evacuations and the sweats.

CASE XI. In Thasus, a woman, of a melancholic turn of mind, from some accidental cause of sorrow, while still going about, became affected with loss of sleep, aversion to food, and had thirst and nausea. She lived near the Pylates, upon the Plain. On the first, at the commencement of night, frights, much talking, despondency, slight fever; in the morning, frequent spasms, and when they ceased, she was incoherent and talked obscurely; pains frequent, great and continued. On the second, in the same state; had no sleep; fever more acute. On the third, the spasms left her; but coma, and disposition to sleep, and again awaked, started up, and could not contain herself; much incoherence; acute fever; on that night a copious sweat all over; apyrexia, slept, quite collected; had a crisis. About the third day, the urine black, thin, substances floating in it generally round, did not fall to the bottom; about the crisis a copious menstruation.

CASE XII. In Larissa, a young unmarried woman was seized with a fever of the acute and ardent type; insomnolency, thirst; tongue sooty and dry; urine of a good color, but thin. On the second, in an uneasy state, did not sleep. On the third, alvine discharges copious, watery, and greenish, and on the following days passed such with relief. On the fourth, passed a small quantity of thin urine, having substances floating towards its surface, which did not subside; was delirious towards night. On the sixth, a great hemorrhage from the nose; a chill, with a copious and hot sweat all over; apyrexia, had a crisis. In the fever, and when it had passed the crisis, the menses took place for the first time, for she was a young woman. Throughout she was oppressed with nausea, and rigors; redness of the face; pain of the eyes; heaviness of the head; she had no relapse, but the fever came to a crisis. The pains were on the even days.

CASE XIII. Apollonius, in Abdera, bore up (under the fever?) for some time, without betaking himself to bed. His viscera were enlarged, and for a considerable time there was a constant pain about the liver, and then he became affected with jaundice; he was flatulent, and of a whitish complexion. Having eaten beef, and drunk unseasonably, he became a little heated at first, and betook himself to bed, and having used large quantities of milk, that of goats and sheep, and both boiled and raw, with a bad diet otherwise, great mischief was occasioned by all these things; for the fever was exacerbated, and of the food taken scarcely any portion worth mentioning was passed from the bowels; the urine was thin and scanty; no sleep; troublesome meteorism; much thirst; disposition to coma; painful swelling of the right hypochondrium; extremities altogether coldish; slight incoherence, forgetfulness of everything he said; he was beside himself. About the fourteenth day after he betook himself to bed, had a rigor, became heated, and was seized with furious delirium; loud cries, much talking, again composed, and then coma came on; afterwards the bowels disordered, with copious, bilious, unmixed, and undigested stools; urine black, scanty, and thin; much restlessness; alvine evacuations of varied characters, either black, scanty, and verdigrisgreen, or fatty, undigested, and acrid; and at times the dejections resembled milk. About the twenty-fourth, enjoyed a calm; other matters in the same state; became somewhat collected; remembered nothing that had happened since he was confined to bed; immediately afterwards became delirious; every symptom rapidly getting worn. About the thirtieth, acute fever; stools copious and thin; was delirious; extremities cold; loss of speech. On the thirty-fourth he died. In this case, as far as I saw, the bowels were disordered; urine thin and black; disposition to coma; insomnolency; extremities cold; delirious throughout. Phrenitis.

CASE XIV. In Cyzicus, a woman who had brought forth twin daughters, after a difficult labor, and in whom the lochial discharge was insufficient, at first was seized with an acute fever, attended with chills; heaviness of the head and neck, with pain; insomnolency from the commencement; she was silent, sullen, and disobedient; urine thin, and devoid of color; thirst, nausea for the most part; bowels irregularly disordered, and again constipated. On the sixth, towards night, talked much incoherently; had no sleep. About the eleventh day was seized with wild delirium, and again became collected; urine black, thin, and again deficient, and of an oily appearance; copious, thin, and disordered evacuations from the bowels. On the fourteenth, frequent convulsions; extremities cold; not in anywise collected; suppression of urine. On the sixteenth loss of speech. On the seventeenth, she died. Phrenitis.

Explanation of the characters. It is probable that death was caused, on the seventeenth day, by the affection of the brain consequent upon her accouchement.

CASE XV. In Thasus, the wife of Dealces, who was lodged upon the Plain, from sorrow was seized with an acute fever, attended with chills. From first to last she wrapped herself up in her bedclothes; still silent, she fumbled, picked, bored, and gathered hairs (from them); tears, and again laughter; no sleep; bowels irritable, but passed nothing; when directed, drank a little; urine thin and scanty; to the touch of the hand the fever was slight; coldness of the extremities. On the ninth, talked much incoherently, and again became composed and silent. On the fourteenth, breathing rare, large, at intervals; and again hurried respiration. On the sixteenth, looseness of the bowels from a stimulant clyster; afterwards she passed her drink, nor could retain anything, for she was completely insensible; skin parched and tense. On the twentieth, much talk, and again became composed; loss of speech; respiration hurried. On the twenty-first she died. Her respiration throughout was rare and large; she was totally insensible; always wrapped up in her bedclothes; either much talk, or completely silent throughout. Phrenitis.

CASE XVI. In Meliboea, a young man having become heated by drinking and much venery, was confined to bed; he was affected with rigors and nausea; insomnolency and absence of thirst. On the first day much faeces passed from the bowels along with a copious flux; and on the following days he passed many watery stools of a green color; urine thin, scanty, and deficient in color; respiration rare, large, at long intervals; softish distention of the hypochondrium, of an oblong form, on both sides; continued palpitation in the epigastric region throughout; passed urine of an oily appearance. On the tenth, he had calm delirium, for he was naturally of an orderly and quiet disposition; skin parched and tense; dejections either copious and thin, or bilious and fatty. On the fourteenth, all the symptoms were exacerbated; he became delirious, and talked much incoherently. On the twentieth, wild delirium, On the twentieth, wild delirium, jactitation, passed no urine; small drinks were retained. On the twenty-fourth he died. Phrenitis.